CLINICAL OUTLINES *for* HEALTH ASSESSMENT

CLINICAL OUTLINES *for* HEALTH ASSESSMENT

June M. Thompson, RN, DrPH

Director of Nursing Education, Research, and Standards,
University of New Mexico Health Sciences Center,
University Hospital,
Albuquerque, New Mexico

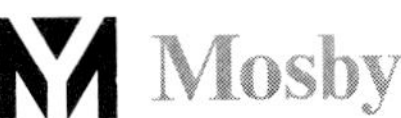

St. Louis Baltimore Boston Carlsbad Chicago Naples New York Philadelphia Portland
London Madrid Mexico City Singapore Sydney Tokyo Toronto Wiesbaden

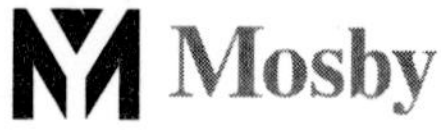

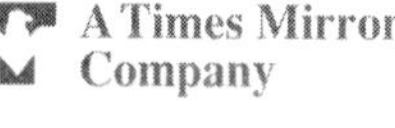

Vice President and Publisher: Nancy L. Coon
Senior Editor: Sally Schrefer
Developmental Editor: Gail Brower
Project Manager: Dana Peick
Production Editor: Jeffrey Patterson
Designer: Renée Duenow
Manufacturing Supervisor: Karen Boehme

Printed in the United States of America
Composition by Top Graphics
Printing/binding by Plus Communications

Mosby–Year Book, Inc.
11830 Westline Industrial Drive
St. Louis, Missouri 63146

International Standard Book Number 0-8151-2578-X

96 97 98 99 00 / 9 8 7 6 5 4 3 2 1

NOTE TO THE READER

This pocket guide to health assessment is designed as a quick reference for students and practitioners. The illustrations and outline format simplify retrieval of material, and the convenient, small size makes the guide easy to carry into the clinical area.

The focus of this guide is the adult client with consideration for the older adult included where appropriate. General pediatric considerations are also included. Part Four presents the development guidelines for the infant and child as well as examination guidelines.

Every attempt has been made to include all of the information necessary to make this a complete yet succinct resource for you. It is the author's sincere hope that you will find this guide helpful in your daily practice.

CONTENTS

PART TWO
Physical Assessment Guide by Body Systems, *22*

CLINICAL OUTLINES *for* HEALTH ASSESSMENT

PART ONE

Health Database

BIOGRAPHIC DATA

The biographic data are collected at the first visit and then updated as changes occur. These data begin to form a picture of the client as a unique individual. See the box on p. 2 for a list of data to be obtained.

REASON FOR SEEKING CARE

Record one brief statement that describes the reason for the client's visit or the client's chief complaint. State this in his or her own words.

PRESENT HEALTH STATUS

Data collected include what clients are doing currently to maintain their health.

- Current health promotion activities: diet, exercise, stress management, meditation, yoga, spiritual or religious groups
- Client's perceived level of health
- Current medications

  Herbal preparations

  Type of drug (prescription, over-the-counter, vitamins, illegal)

  Prescribed by whom

  When first prescribed

  Reason for prescription

  Amount of medication and frequency per day

  Effectiveness of medication

Biographic Data Summary

Name
Address and telephone number
Birth date
Birthplace (important when born in a foreign country)
Race (physical features such as skin color, bone structure, or blood group that are genetically determined)
Culture (pattern of behavioral responses shaped by values, beliefs, norms, and practices)
Religion
Marital status
Family or significant others living in the home
Social security number
Occupation
Contact person
Advance directive (decisions about end-of-life care)
Durable power of attorney for health care
Source of referral
Usual source of health care
Type of health insurance

ANALYSIS OF A SYMPTOM

When a client seeks relief from a specific problem, obtain the following data for symptom analysis:

Location

Where are the symptoms?

- Is the location in a specific area? Vague and generalized? Does the symptom radiate?

Quality

Describe the characteristics of the symptom.

- Describe the sensation: stabbing, dull, aching, throbbing, nagging, sharp, squeezing, itching.
- Describe the drainage: color, texture, composition, appearance, and odor.
- Was the onset slow? Abrupt? Noticeable to others?
- Was the symptom intermittent or continuous?
- How has the symptom interrupted your life (e.g., sleeping, eating, working, activities at home or school)?

Quantity

Describe the severity of the symptom.

- Describe the size, extent, number, or amount (e.g., of lesion, rash, blister, discharge).
- Was the symptom so severe that it interrupted your activities?
- On a scale of 1 to 10, with 10 being most severe, how would you rate your symptom?

Chronology

When did the symptom start?

- Ask specific date, time, and day of the week.
- How many times a day, week, month does the symptom occur?
- How did the client feel between episodes of the symptom?

Setting

Where are you when the symptom occurs?

- Does anyone else with whom you have been in contact have a similar symptom?
- Are there psychologic or physical factors in the environment that may be causing the symptom (e.g., stress, smoke, or chemicals)?

Associated Manifestations

Do other symptoms occur at the same time?

- What effects does the symptom have on body function? Activities? Appetite?

Alleviating Factors

- What home remedies have you tried?
- What medications have you tried (over-the-counter and prescription)?
- Are there certain body positions that relieve the symptom?

Aggravating Factors

- Is the symptom associated with an activity (e.g., walking, climbing stairs, eating, a body position)?

HEALTH HISTORY

Health history is important, since past illnesses may have some effect on the client's current health needs or problems. The following categories of data are included:

- *Allergies:* food, drugs, environmental factors, contact substances
- *Childhood illnesses:* measles, mumps, rubella, chicken pox, pertussis, haemophilus influenza, streptococcal throat infection, otitis media. (Ask if there were complications in later years, such as rheumatic fever or glomerulonephritis that can occur after streptococcal throat infection.)
- *Surgeries:* type, date, outcome
- *Hospitalizations:* illnesses, dates, outcome
- *Injuries:* fractures, lacerations, loss of consciousness, burns, penetrating wounds
- *Chronic illnesses:* diabetes, hypertension, heart disease, sickle cell anemia, cancer, seizures, chronic obstructive pulmonary disease, arthritis. Ask how often the illness interferes with daily activities.
- *Immunizations:* tetanus, diphtheria, pertussis; mumps, rubella; poliomyelitis; hepatitis B; influenza, pneumococcus pneumonia, varicella, and for foreign-born clients, bacillus-Calmette-Guerin (BCG)
- *Last examinations:* physical, dental, vision, hearing, ECG, chest radiograph, skin test for tuberculosis; for women: Papanicolaou (Pap) smear, mammogram
- *Obstetric history:* number of pregnancies (gravidity, number of births [parity], and number of abortions or miscarriages). For each birth, document the course of pregnancy, labor, type of delivery [vaginal or cesarean section], weight of neonate, and postpartum course.

FAMILY HISTORY

Family history of the client's blood relatives, spouse, and children is obtained to identify any illnesses of a genetic, familial, or environmental nature that might affect the client's current or future health. Trace back at least two generations to maternal and paternal parents and grandparents. Also include siblings, uncles, and aunts. Ask about health information of significant others, sexual partners, and roommates if relevant to the client's health. Questions about the health of family members should include the following:

- Alzheimer's disease
- Cancer (all types)
- Diabetes mellitus
- Mental diseases
- Developmental delay
- Alcoholism
- Heart disease
- Hypertension
- Seizures
- Emotional problems
- Endocrine diseases (specify)
- Sickle cell anemia
- Kidney disease
- Cerebrovascular accident

REVIEW OF SYSTEMS

General Health Status

- Fatigue, weakness
- Sleep patterns
- Weight, unexplained loss or gain
- Self-rating of overall health status

Integumentary System

Skin

- Skin disease, problems, lesions (wounds, sores, ulcers)
- Skin growths, tumors, masses
- Excessive dryness, sweating, odors
- Pigmentation changes or discolorations
- Rashes
- Pruritus (itching)
- Frequent bruising
- Texture or temperature change
- Scalp itching
- Health promotion *(HP):* Amount of sun exposure, including tanning bed use; use of sun screen; skin self-examination

Hair (refers to all body hair, not just head and pubic area)

- Changes in amount, texture, character, distribution
- Alopecia (loss of hair)
- HP: Use of dyes, permanent waves, or other chemicals

Nails

- Changes in texture, color, shape
- HP: Type and frequency of nail care

Head

- Headache (characteristics, frequency, location and type of pain, duration)
- Past significant trauma
- Vertigo (dizziness)
- Syncope (brief lapse of consciousness)

Eyes

- Discharge (describe)
- Pruritus
- Lacrimation (excessive tearing)
- Pain in eyeball
- Visual disturbances such as blind spots (floaters), halos around lights, or flashing lights
- Swelling around eyes
- Redness
- Cataracts
- History of glaucoma
- Unusual sensations or twitching
- Vision changes (generalized or vision field)
- Use of corrective or prosthetic devices
- Diplopia (double vision)
- Blurring vision
- Photophobia (increased sensitivity to light)
- Difficulty reading
- Interferences with activities of daily living
- HP: Use of protective eyewear

Ears

- Pain
- Cerumen (wax)
- Infection, earache
- Discharge (describe)
- Hearing changes (describe)
- Use of prosthetic devices
- Increased sensitivity to environmental noises
- Vertigo (dizziness, unable to maintain balance)
- Tinnitus (ringing or cracking)
- Interference with activities of daily living

Nose, Nasopharynx, and Paranasal Sinuses

- Discharge (describe, seasonal occurrence)
- Epistaxis (nose bleed)
- Sneezing
- Obstruction
- Sinus pain
- Postnasal drip
- Change in ability to smell
- Snoring
- Pain over sinuses

Mouth and Oropharynx

- Sore throat (describe)
- Tongue or mouth lesion (abscess, sore, ulcer)
- Bleeding gums
- Voice changes or hoarseness
- Use of prosthetic devices (dentures, bridges)
- Altered taste
- Dysphagia (difficulty swallowing)
- Difficulty chewing
- HP: Frequency and kind of dental hygiene

Neck

- Lymph node enlargement
- Swelling or masses
- Pain or tenderness
- Limitation of movement
- Stiffness

Breasts

- Nipple discharge (describe)
- Changes in nipples
- Lumps, masses, dimples
- Unusual characteristics
- HP: Breast self-examination (frequency, method)

Cardiovascular System

Heart

- Palpitations
- Heart murmur
- Hypertension
- Chest pain (describe quality, duration)
- Dyspnea (shortness of breath)
- Orthopnea (person must sit to breathe)

- Paroxysmal nocturnal dyspnea (periodic dyspnea during sleep)
- HP: Monitoring of fat in diet; regular exercise

Peripheral vasculature

- Coldness, numbness
- Discoloration
- Peripheral edema
- Varicose veins
- Intermittent claudication (leg pain with exercise that ceases with rest)
- Paresthesia (abnormal sensations)
- Leg color change
- HP:
  Use support hose if work involves standing
  Avoid crossing legs at the knees
  Perform exercise patterns

Respiratory System

- Cold
- Cough, nonproductive or productive (describe sputum)
- Hemoptysis (coughing up blood)
- Dyspnea (shortness of breath)
- Night sweats
- Wheezing
- Stridor (abnormal, high-pitched, musical sound)
- Pain on inspiration or expiration
- Smoker; exposure to smoke

Gastrointestinal System

- Change in taste
- Thirst
- Indigestion or pain associated with eating
- Pyrosis (burning sensation in esophagus and stomach with sour eructation [belching])
- Dyspepsia (heartburn or bloating)
- Nausea or vomiting (describe)
- Hematemesis (vomiting blood)
- Appetite changes
- Food intolerance
- Abdominal pain (describe)
- Jaundice (yellowish color to skin and sclera)

- Ascites (abnormal intraperitoneal fluid accumulation)
- Bowel habits (frequency)
- Flatus
- Constipation
- Diarrhea
- Dyschezia (constipation resulting from habitual neglect in responding to stimulus to defecate)
- Changes in stools (color, consistency)
- Hemorrhoids (pain, rectal bleeding)
- Use of digestive or evacuation aids (type, frequency)
- HP: Type of diet; compare diet with food pyramid (see p. 17)

Urinary System

- Characteristics of urine (color, contents)
- Hesitancy
- Urinary frequency (in 24-hour period)
- Urgency
- Change in urinary stream
- Nocturia (excessive urination at night)
- Dysuria (painful urination)
- Flank pain (posterior portion of body between ribs and ileum)
- Hematuria
- Suprapubic pain
- Dribbling or incontinence
- Polyuria (excessive excretion of urine)
- HP: Amount of water drunk daily
- Females—measures to prevent urinary tract infections

Genitalia

General

- Lesions
- Discharges
- Odors
- Pain, burning, pruritus
- Satisfaction with sexual activity
- Sexual preference
- Number of partners
- Method of birth control
- Infertility

- HP: Methods of protection from unwanted pregnancy and sexually transmitted diseases

Men

- Impotence
- Testicular masses or pain
- Prostate problems
- Change in sex drive
- HP: Penis and scrotum self-examination practices

Women

- Menstrual history (date of onset, last menstrual period, length of cycle)
- Amenorrhea (absent menstruation)
- Menorrhagia (excessive menstruation)
- Dysmenorrhea (painful menstruation)
- Metrorrhagia (irregular menstruation)
- Dysparenunia (pain during intercourse)
- Postcoital bleeding (bleeding after intercourse)
- Pelvic pain
- HP: Genitalia self-examination, Pap smears

Musculoskeletal System

Muscles

- Twitching, cramping, pain
- Weakness

Bones and joints

- Joint swelling, pain, redness, stiffness (time of day, duration)
- Joint deformity
- Crepitus (noise with joint movement)
- Limitations in joint range of motion
- Interference with activities of daily living

Back

- Pain
- Limitations in joint range of motion
- Interference with activities of daily living
- HP: Amount and kind of exercise per week

Central Nervous System

- History of central nervous system disease (specify with examples)

- Fainting episodes or loss of consciousness
- Seizures (characteristics, how treated)
- Dysphasia (impaired speech)
- Dysarthria (poorly articulated speech)
- Cognitive changes
  Inability to remember (recent vs. dated)
  Disorientation to time, place, person
  Hallucinations

Motor-gait

- Loss of coordinated movements
- Ataxia (balance problems)
- Paralysis (partial vs. complete)
- Paresis
- Tic, tremor, spasm
- Interference with activities of daily living

Sensory

- Paresthesia (abnormal sensations [e.g., "pins and needles," tingling, numbness])
- Anesthesia (absent sensation, location)
- Pain (describe)

Endocrine System

- Changes in skin pigmentation or texture
- Changes in or abnormal hair distribution
- Sudden or unexplained change in height or weight
- Intolerance of heat or cold
- Hormone therapy
- Presence of secondary sex characteristics
- Polydipsia (excessive thirst)
- Polyphagia (excessive hunger)
- Polyuria (excessive urine output)
- Anorexia (decreased appetite)
- Weakness

PSYCHOSOCIAL STATUS

Psychologic and sociologic data are important aspects of a health history. The following is an outline of information to be obtained:

- General statement of client's feelings about self
  Degree of satisfaction in interpersonal relationships
  Client's position in home relationships

Most significant relationship
Community activities
Work or school relationships
Family cohesiveness

- Activities

General description of work, leisure, and rest distribution
Hobbies and methods of relaxation
Family demands
Ability to accomplish all that is desired during period (day, week)

- Cultural or religious practices
- Occupational history

Jobs held in past
Current employer
Education preparation
Satisfaction with present and past employment

- Recent changes or stresses in client's life (e.g., divorce, moving, new job, family illness, new baby, financial stress)
- Coping strategies for stressful situations
- Change in personality, behavior, mood

Feelings of anxiety or nervousness
Feelings of depression (e.g., insomnia, crying, fearfulness, marked irritability or anger)
Use of medications or other techniques during times of anxiety, stress, or depression

- Habits

Alcohol or drugs

- Type of alcohol or drugs
- Frequency per week
- Pattern over past 5 years; 1 year
- Drinking or drug consumption variances when anxious, stressed, or depressed
- Driving or other dangerous activities while under the influence
- High-risk groups: sharing or using unsterilized needles and syringes

Smoking

- Kind (cigarette, cigar, pipe)
- Amount per day
- Pattern over 5 years; 1 year
- Smoking variances when anxious or stressed
- Desire to quit smoking

- Exposure to second-hand smoke

Coffee and tea

- Amount per day
- Pattern over 5 years; 1 year
- Consumption variances when anxious or stressed
- Physiologic effects

Other

- Overeating, sporadic eating, or fasting
- Nail biting
- "Street drug" use

- Financial status

  Sources of income

  Adequacy of income

  Recent changes in resources or expenditures

ENVIRONMENTAL HEALTH

An outline of data to be obtained for the environmental health portion of the history includes the following:

- General statement of the client's assessment of environmental safety and comfort
- Hazards of employment (inhalants, noise, heavy lifting, machinery, psychologic stress)
- Hazards in the home (concern about fire, smoke detector, stairs to climb, inadequate heat, open gas heaters, pest control, violent behaviors, loud sound systems including earphones)
- Hazards in the neighborhood or community (noise, water and air pollution, heavy traffic on surrounding streets, overcrowding, violence, firearms, sale or use of "street drugs")
- Hazards of travel (use of seat belts, motorcycle or bicycle helmets)

  Travel outside the United States (when and which countries visited, length of stay)

SAFETY ASSESSMENT

Use the following optional assessment if the client is disabled or has difficulty with activities of daily living:

A. Gait and balance problems
   1. Slippery or irregular surfaces
   2. Obstruction or clutter

3. Steep or dark stairs
4. Slippery bathtub
5. Shoes without support
6. Climbing or use of ladder
7. Clothing too long
8. Walking in busy traffic areas

B. Decreased vision
1. Insufficient illumination in home
2. Glare from polished floor
3. Missing the bottom step
4. Bifocals
5. Medication error

C. Decreased sensation to pain or heat
1. Hot bath water
2. Heating pads or hot water bottle

D. Other
1. Fire hazards
2. Driving or motor vehicle crashes

ACTIVITIES OF DAILY LIVING (ADL) ASSESSMENT

Use this optional assessment if client is disabled.

A. Self-care
1. Dressing, undressing, clothing
   a. Keeping clothes in good repair (mending)
   b. Access to clothes
   c. Getting into and out of underwear (bra, girdle, underpants, pantyhose, stockings, garter belt)
   d. Putting on and removing pants
   e. Getting arms in sleeves
   f. Managing zippers, buttons, snaps (especially in back), ties
   g. Putting on socks, shoes; tying laces
   h. Applying prostheses (e.g., glasses, hearing aids)
2. Grooming and hygiene
   a. Washing, drying, brushing hair
   b. Brushing teeth

c. Cleaning and putting in dentures
d. Shaving
e. Nail care: feet and hands
f. Applying makeup
g. Preparing bath water and testing temperature
h. Getting into and out of tub, shower
i. Reaching and cleaning all body parts

3. Elimination
a. Position altered for urination or sitting on toilet
b. Ability to wipe self
c. Lowering onto and rising from toilet

B. Mobility
1. Difficulty climbing or descending stairs: Is bedroom/bathroom on upper level? How many stairs/flights to apartment or house?
2. Sitting up, rising from bed
3. Lowering to or rising from chair
4. Walking: short and long distances (describe necessity for walking)
5. Opening doors
6. Reaching items in cupboards
7. Necessity for lifting: any difficulty

C. Communication
1. Dialing telephone
2. Reading numbers
3. Hearing over telephone
4. Answering door
5. Immediate access to help from neighbors

D. Eating
1. Access to market
2. Preparing food (opening cans, packages; using stove; reaching dishes, pots, utensils)
3. Handling knife, fork, spoon; cutting meat
4. Getting food to mouth
5. Chewing, swallowing

E. Housekeeping, laundry, house upkeep
1. Making bed
2. Sweeping, mopping floors
3. Dusting
4. Cleaning dishes
5. Cleaning tub, bathroom
6. Picking up clutter (to patient's satisfaction)

7. Taking out trash, garbage
8. Use of basement: stairs, cleaning
9. Laundry facilities: in home or near residence, washtub, clothesline
10. Yard care: garden, bushes, grass
11. Other home maintenance concerns (e.g., access to fuse box, storm windows, furnace filters, painting)

F. Medications
   1. Large number of prescriptions
   2. Difficulty remembering
   3. Ability to see labels or directions
   4. Medications kept in one area

G. Access to community
   1. Bus line
   2. Walking
   3. Driving (self or service from others)
   4. Church, dry cleaning, drugstore, bank, health care facility, dentist, other community agencies

H. Other
   1. Caring for spouse/relative/companion
   2. Financial management: able to write checks, make payments, cash checks
   3. Care of pet(s)

NUTRITION ASSESSMENT

Screening tools for dietary assessment include food recall for 24 hours, food frequency, food checklists, diet records, and nutrition questionnaires. Clients also should be interviewed regarding food allergies or intolerances to specific foods. Below is one example of a nutrition questionnaire.

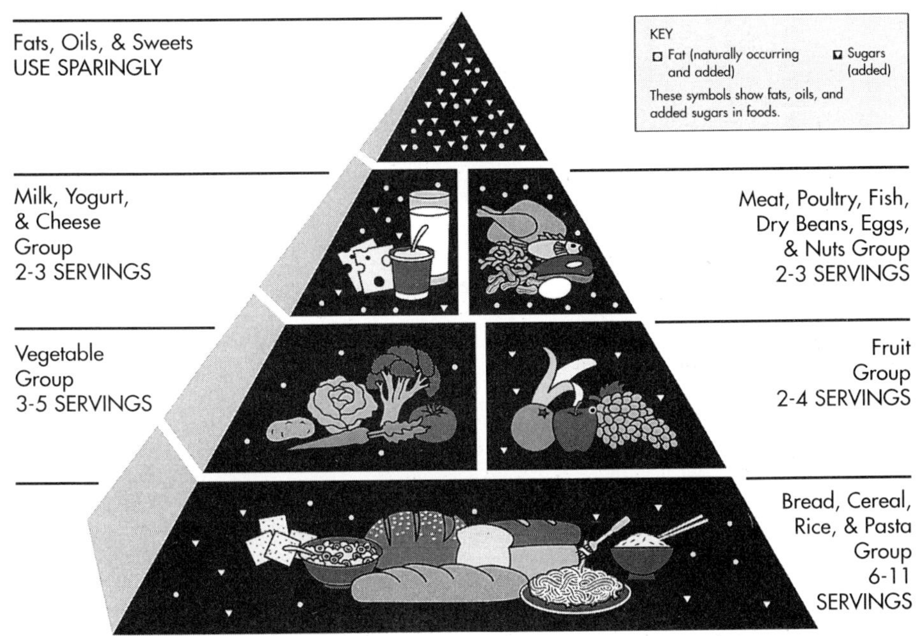
Fats, Oils, & Sweets
USE SPARINGLY
KEY
Fat (naturally occurring and added)
Sugars (added)
These symbols show fats, oils, and added sugars in foods.
Milk, Yogurt, & Cheese Group
2-3 SERVINGS
Meat, Poultry, Fish, Dry Beans, Eggs, & Nuts Group
2-3 SERVINGS
Vegetable Group
3-5 SERVINGS
Fruit Group
2-4 SERVINGS
Bread, Cereal, Rice, & Pasta Group
6-11 SERVINGS

Nutrition Questionnaire

What you eat and some of the lifestyle choices you make can affect your nutrition and health now and in the future. Please answer these questions by circling the answers that apply to you.

Eating Behavior

1. Are you frequently bothered by any of the following? (Circle all that apply):
   Nausea Vomiting Heartburn Constipation
2. Do you skip meals at least 3 times a week? No Yes
3. Do you try to limit the amount or kind of food you eat to control your weight? No Yes
4. Are you on a special diet now? No Yes
5. Do you avoid any foods for health or religious reasons? No Yes

Food Resources

6. Do you have a working stove? No Yes
   Do you have a working refrigerator No Yes

12. Which of these foods did you eat yesterday? (Circle all that apply):

Cheese	Pizza	Macaroni and cheese
Yogurt	Cereal with milk	

Other foods made with cheese (such as tacos, enchiladas, lasagna, cheeseburgers)

Corn	Potatoes	Sweet potatoes
Green salad	Carrots	Collard greens
Spinach	Turnip greens	Broccoli
Green beans	Green peas	Other vegetables
Apples	Bananas	Berries
Grapefruit	Melon	Oranges
Peaches	Other fruit	
Meat	Fish	Chicken
Eggs	Peanut butter	Nuts
Seeds	Dried beans	
Cold cuts	Hot dog	Bacon
Sausage	Cake	Cookies
Doughnut	Pastry	Chips
French fries		

7. Do you sometimes run out of food before you are able to buy more? No Yes
8. Can you afford to eat the way you should? No Yes
9. Are you receiving any food assistance now? (Circle all that apply) No Yes

   Food stamps School breakfast School lunch
   WIC Donated food/commodities CSFP
   Food from a food pantry, soup kitchen, or food bank
10. Do you feel you need help in obtaining food? No Yes

Food and Drink

11. Which of these did you drink yesterday? (Circle all that apply):

    Soft drinks Coffee Tea
    Fruit drink Orange juice Grapefruit juice
    Other juices Milk Kool-Aid
    Beer Wine Alcoholic drinks
    Water Other beverages (list) ________

    Other deep-fried foods, such as fried chicken or egg rolls
    Bread Rolls Rice Tortillas
    Cereal Noodles Spaghetti
    Were any of these whole grain? No Yes
13. Is the way you ate yesterday the way you usually eat? No Yes

Lifestyle

14. Do you exercise for at least 30 minutes on a regular basis (3 times a week or more)? No Yes
15. Do you ever smoke cigarettes or use smokeless tobacco? No Yes
16. Do you ever drink beer, wine, liquor, or any other alcoholic beverages? No Yes
17. Which of these do you take? (Circle all that apply):

    Prescribed drugs or medications
    Any over-the-counter products (such as aspirin, Tylenol, antacids, or vitamins)
    Street drugs (such as marijuana, speed, downers, crack, or heroin)

Details of the Food Pyramid

FOOD GROUP	SUGGESTED DAILY SERVINGS	WHAT COUNTS AS A SERVING?
Breads, cereals, and other grain products Whole-grain Enriched	**6-11** servings from entire group (Include several servings of whole-grain products daily.)	• 1 slice of bread • ½ hamburger bun or english muffin • 1 small roll, biscuit, or muffin • 3 to 4 small or 2 large crackers • ½ cup cooked cereal, rice, pasta • 1 ounce of ready-to-eat breakfast cereal
Fruits Citrus, melon, berries Other fruits	**2-4** servings from entire group	• 1 whole fruit such as a medium apple, banana, or orange • 1 grapefruit half • 1 melon wedge • ¾ cup of juice • ½ cup of berries • ½ cup cooked or canned fruit • ½ cup dried fruit
Vegetables Dark-green leafy Deep-yellow Dry beans/peas (legumes) Starchy Other vegetables	**3-5** servings from entire group (Include all types regularly: use dark-green leafy vegetables and dry beans and peas several times a week.)	• ½ cup of cooked vegetables • ½ cup of chopped raw vegetables • 1 cup of leafy raw vegetables, such as lettuce or spinach

Meat, poultry, fish and alternates (eggs, dry beans and peas, nuts and seeds)	**2-3** servings from entire group	Amounts should total 5 to 7 ounces of cooked lean meat, poultry, or fish a day. Count 1 egg, ½ cup cooked beans, or 2 tablespoons peanut butter as 1 ounce of meat.
Milk, cheese, and yogurt	**2** servings from entire group (3 servings for women who are pregnant or breast-feeding and for teens; 4 servings for teens who are pregnant or breast-feeding)	• 1 cup of milk • 8 ounces of yogurt • 1½ ounces of natural cheese • 2 ounces of process cheese
Fats, sweets, and alcoholic beverages	Avoid too many fats and sweets. If you drink alcoholic beverages, do so in moderation.	

From Oklahoma Diet Manuel, ed 9, 1993.

PART TWO

Physical Assessment Guide by Body Systems

GENERAL ASSESSMENT

- Temperature
- All pulses
- Respirations: rate, characteristics
- Blood pressure: both arms (sitting, standing, lying)
- Height
- Weight

SKIN, HAIR, AND NAILS

Skin

- Inspect the skin for the following:
  Appearance
  Color
  Pigmentation
  Vascularity
  Bruising
- Inspect and palpate the skin for the following:
  Texture
  Lesions
- Palpate the skin for the following:
  Temperature
  Moisture
  Mobility
  Turgor

Hair

- Inspect and palpate the scalp and the hair for the following:
  Surface characteristics
  Hair distribution
  Texture
  Quantity
  Color
- Inspect the facial and body hair for the following:
  Distribution
  Quantity
  Texture

Lesion Characteristics to Be Noted During Examination

- Note the **location and distribution** of the lesion. Is the lesion generalized over the entire body or section of the body, or is it localized to a specific area such as around the waist, under a piece of jewelry, or just in the hair?
- Describe the **color** of the lesion, and describe how this lesion may be different in color from other lesions noted on the body (e.g., a mole or freckle). Has the patient noticed a change in the color of the lesion?
- What is the **pattern** of the lesion? Are the lesions clustered? Are they in a line? How does the patient describe the development of the pattern of the lesion?
- What are the **edges** of the lesion like? Is the edge of the lesion regular or irregular? Has the patient noticed a change in the shape of the lesion?
- Is the lesion **flat, raised, or sunken?**
- What is the current **size** of the lesion? Measure using a centimeter ruler. Has the patient noticed a change in the size of the lesion?
- What are the **characteristics** of the lesion? Is it hard, soft, or fluid-filled? If there is an exudate, what is the color of the drainage fluid? Does the exudate have an odor? Note both the color and odor if present. Has the patient noticed a change in either the characteristics or drainage of the lesion? If so, how and when?

PRIMARY SKIN LESIONS

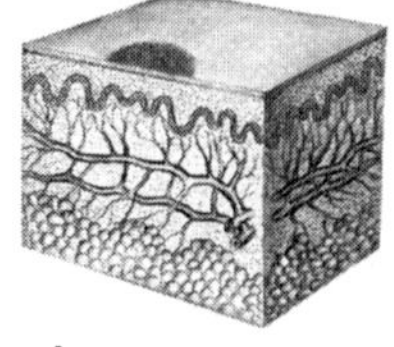

Macule
Flat, nonpalpable, circumscribed, less than 1 cm in diameter, brown, red, purple, white, or tan

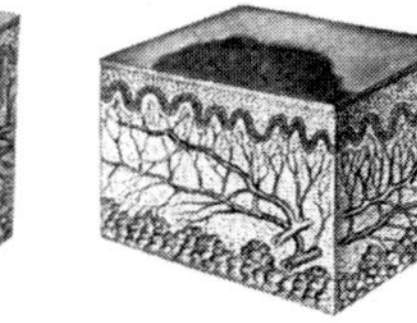

Patch
Flat, nonpalpable, irregularly shaped (macule greater than 1 cm in diameter)

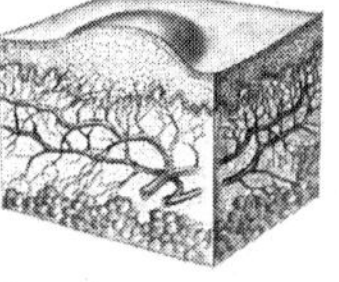

Papule
Elevated, palpable, firm, circumscribed, less than 1 cm in diameter, brown, red, pink, tan, or bluish red

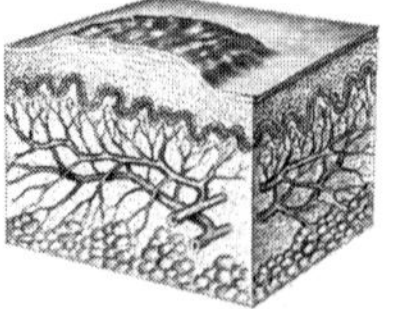

Plaque
Elevated, flat topped, firm, rough (superficial papule greater than 1 cm in diameter, may be coalesced papules)

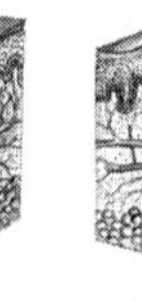

Wheal
Elevated, irregularly shaped area of cutaneous edema, solid, transient, changing, variable diameter, pale pink

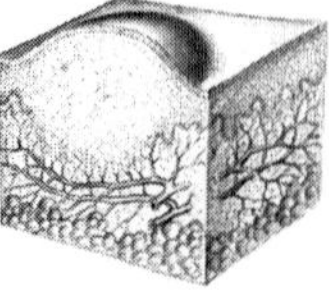

Nodule
Elevated, firm, circumscribed, palpable, deeper in dermis than papule, 1 to 2 cm in diameter

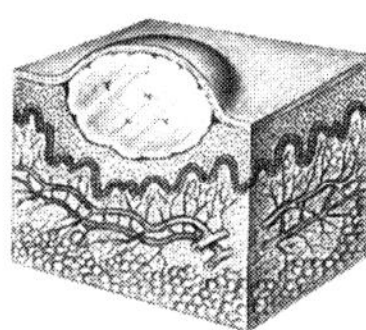

Tumor
Elevated, solid, may or may not be clearly demarcated, greater than 2 cm in diameter, may or may not vary from skin color

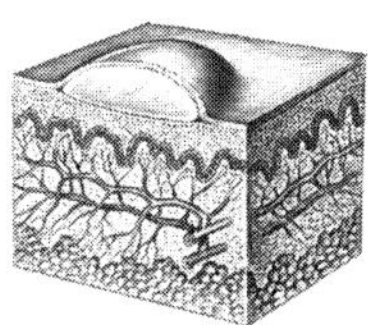

Vesicle
Elevated, circumscribed, superficial, filled with serous fluid, less than 1 cm in diameter

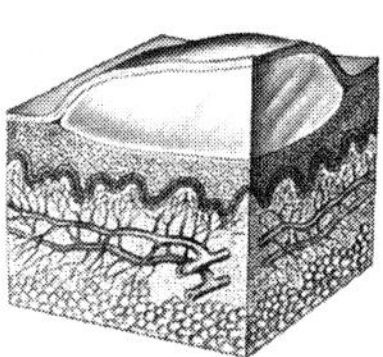

Bulla
Vesicle greater than 1 cm in diameter

Pustule
Elevated, superficial (similar to vesicle but filled with purulent fluid)

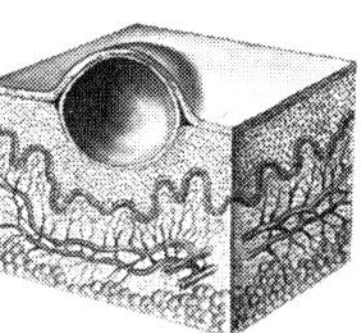

Cyst
Elevated, circumscribed, palpable, encapsulated, filled with liquid or semisolid material

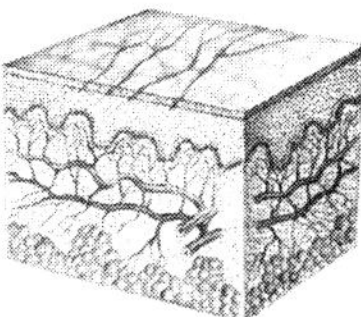

Telangiectasia
Fine, irregular red line produced by dilation of capillary

SECONDARY SKIN LESIONS

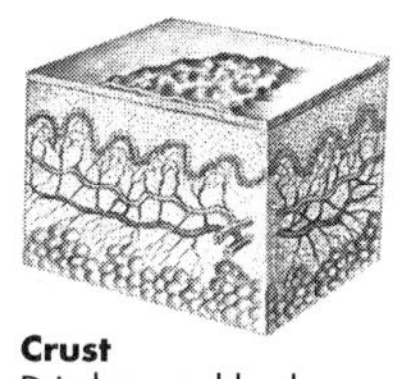

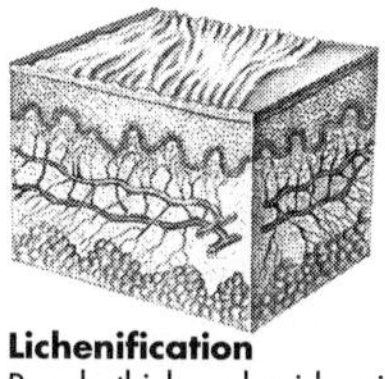

Scale
Heaped-up keratinized cells, flaky exfoliation, irregular, thick or thin, dry or oily, varied size, silver, white, or tan

Crust
Dried serum, blood, or purulent exudate, slightly elevated, size varies, brown, red, black, tan, or straw

Lichenification
Rough, thickened epidermis, accentuated skin markings from rubbing or irritation, often involves flexor aspect of extremity

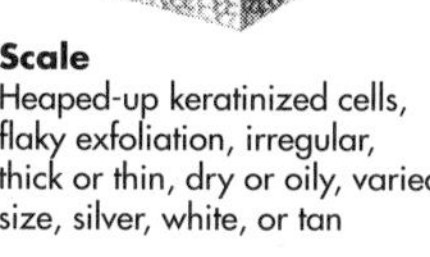

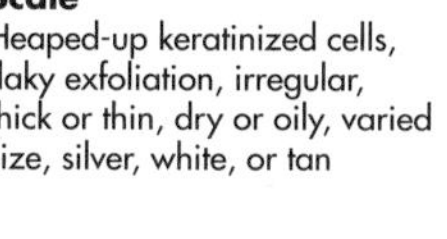

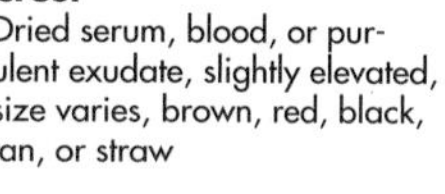

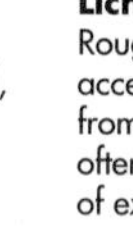

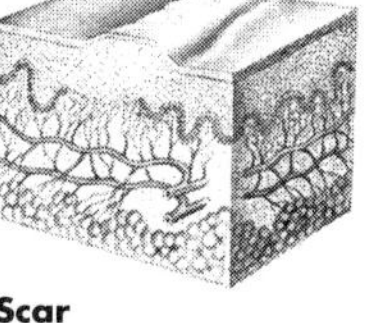

Scar
Thin to thick fibrous tissue replacing injured dermis, irregular, pink, red, or white, may be atrophic or hypertrophic

Keloid
Irregularly shaped, elevated, progressively enlarging scar, grows beyond boundaries of wound, from excessive collagen formation during healing

Excoriation
Loss of epidermis, linear or hollowed-out crusted area, dermis exposed

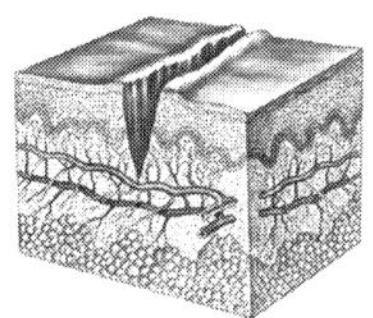

Fissure
Linear crack or break from epidermis to dermis, small, deep, red

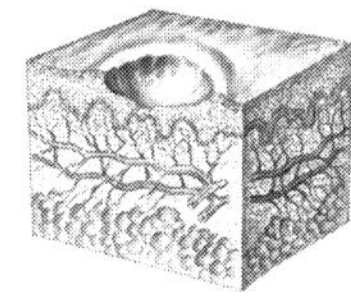

Erosion
Loss of all or part of epidermis, depressed, moist, glistening (follows rupture of vesicle or bulla, larger than fissure)

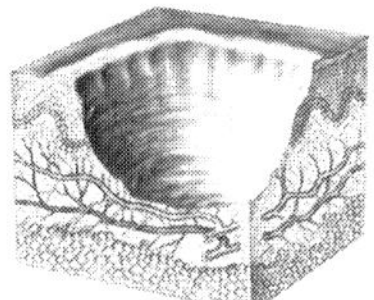

Ulcer
Loss of epidermis and dermis, concave, size varies, exudative, red, or reddish blue

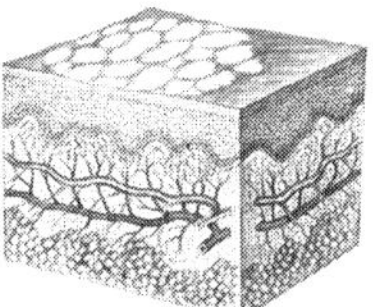

Atrophy
Thinning of skin surface and loss of skin markings, skin translucent and paperlike

Nails

- Inspect and palpate the nails for the following:
  Shape
  Contour
  Consistency
  Color
  Thickness
  Cleanliness

LYMPHATIC SYSTEM

The lymphatic system is examined region by region during the examination of related body parts (head and neck, breast and axilla, arm, and groin).

Head and Neck

(Preauricular, cervical chain, and supraclavicular nodes)

- Inspect the superficial nodes for the following:
  Edema
  Erythema
  Red streaks
- Palpate the nodes for the following:

Size
Consistency
Mobility
Borders
Tenderness
Warmth

Axillary and Breast

- Palpate the nodes for the following:
  Size
  Consistency
  Mobility
  Borders
  Tenderness
  Warmth

Arm

(Epitrochlear)

- Palpate the nodes for the following:
  Size
  Consistency
  Mobility

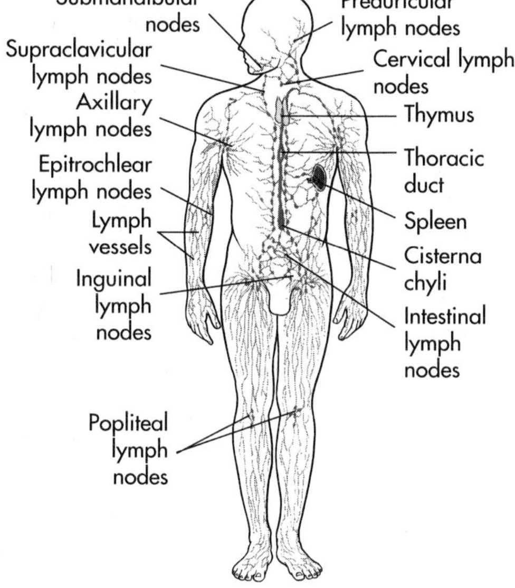

The major organs and vessels of the lymphatic system. (Modified from Thibodeau and Patton.)

Borders
Tenderness
Warmth

Groin

(Inguinal)

- Palpate the nodes for the following:
  Size
  Consistency
  Mobility
  Borders
  Tenderness
  Warmth

HEAD AND NECK

Head

- Inspect the head for the following:
  Facial features
  Appropriateness of facial expression
  Head size
- Palpate the skull for the following:
  Contour and intactness

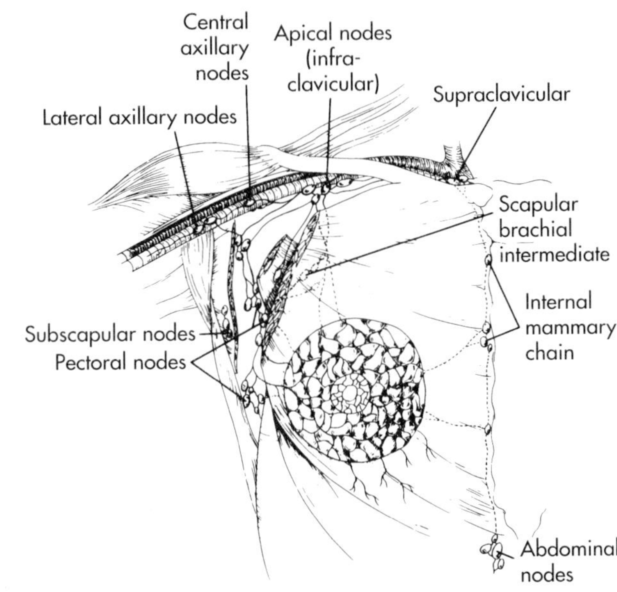

Lymphatic drainage of the breast.

Tenderness

- Inspect and palpate the face and jaw for the following:
  Size
  Symmetry
  Intactness
  Tenderness

Neck

- Inspect and palpate the neck for the following:
  Positioning in relation to the head
  Symmetry of muscles
  Range of motion
  Pain with movement
  Evidence of edema or enlargement of the thyroid area
  Deviation of the trachea

Thyroid

- Palpate the thyroid for the following:
  Size
  Shape

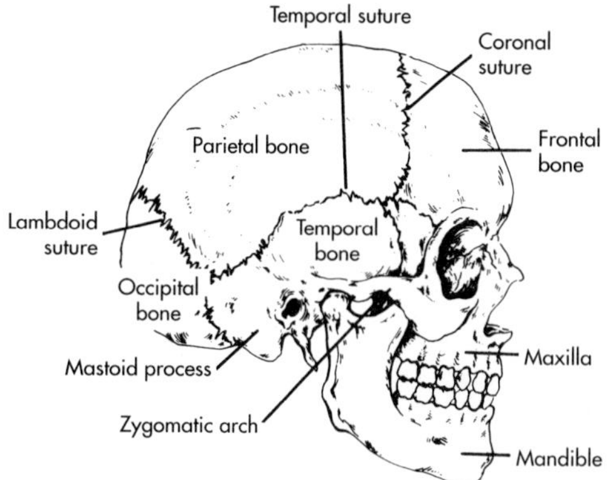

Anatomic landmarks of the skull.

Consistency
Tenderness
Presence of nodules or enlargement

NOSE, PARANASAL SINUSES, MOUTH, AND OROPHARYNX

Nose and Paranasal Sinuses

- Inspect and palpate the nose for the following:
  General appearance and symmetry
  Discharge
  Tenderness
- Evaluate the olfactory nerve for intactness.
- Inspect the internal nasal cavity for patency.
- Inspect and palpate the paranasal sinuses for the following:
  Swelling
  Tenderness or bogginess

Mouth and Oropharynx

- Palpate the temporomandibular joint for tenderness or discomfort.
- Note the breath for odor.
- Inspect the lips for the following:
  Color
  Symmetry
  Moisture
  Texture
- Inspect the teeth for the following:
  Alignment
  Number
  Color
  Surface characteristics
  Stability
- Inspect the oral cavity and buccal mucosa for the following:
  Color
  Symmetry
  Texture
- Inspect and palpate the tongue for the following:
  Movement
  Symmetry
  Color

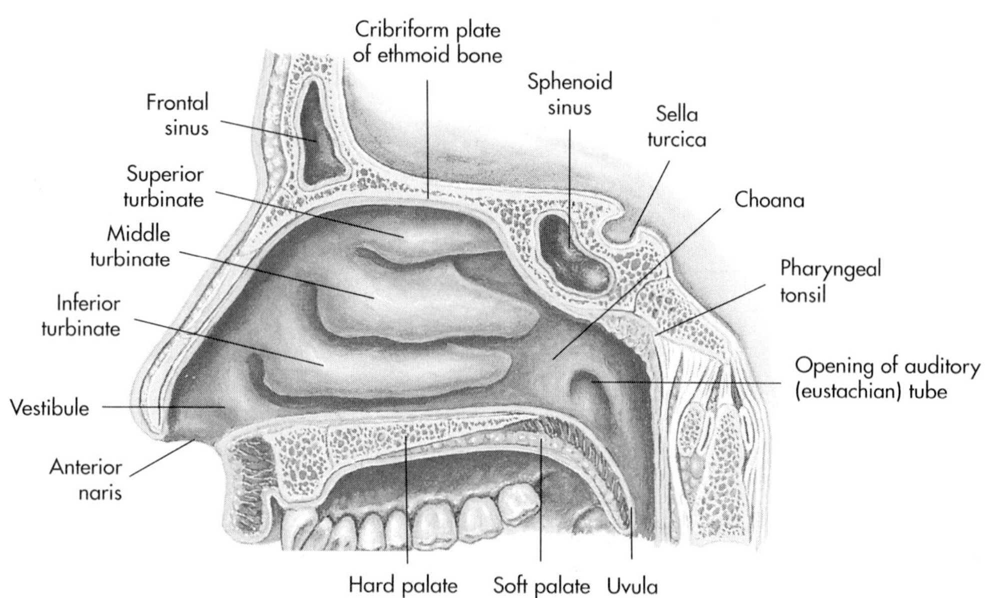

Cross-sectional view of the anatomic structures of the nose and nasopharynx. (From Seidel et al, 1995.)

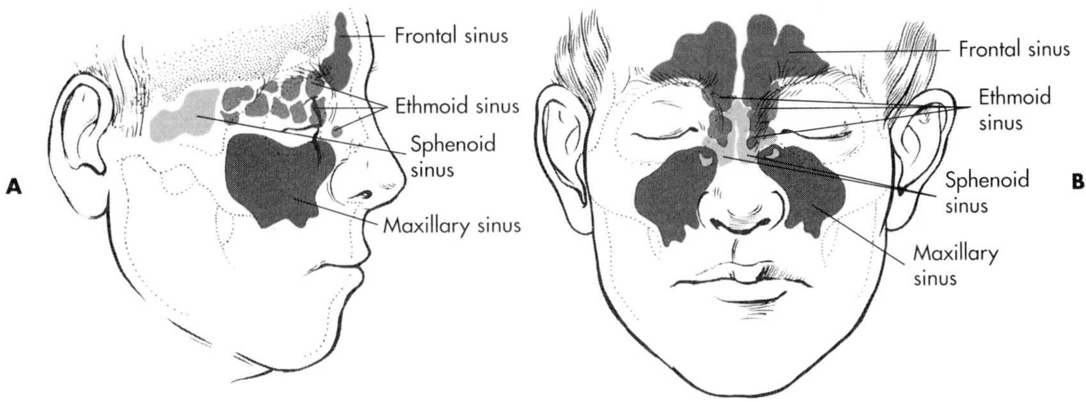

Paranasal sinues. **A,** Side view. **B,** Front view. (From Seeley, Stephens, and Tate, 1995.)

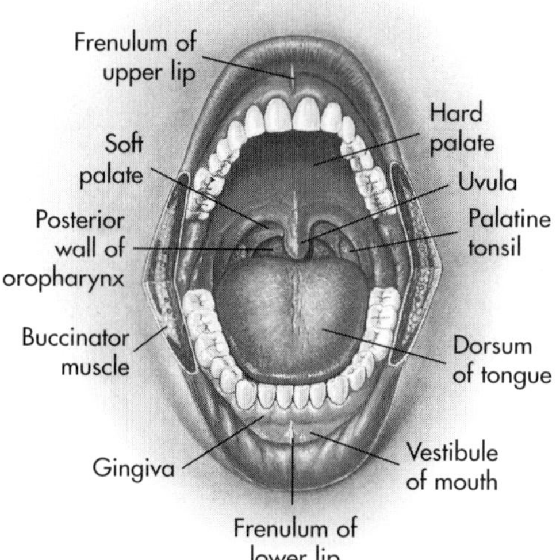

Anatomic structures of the oral cavity. (From Seidel et al, 1995.)

Ulceration
Surface characteristics
Lesions

- Inspect the hard and soft palates for the following:
  Texture
  Color
  Surface characteristics
- Inspect the posterior wall of the pharynx and the tonsils for the following:
  Color
  Surface characteristics
  Texture

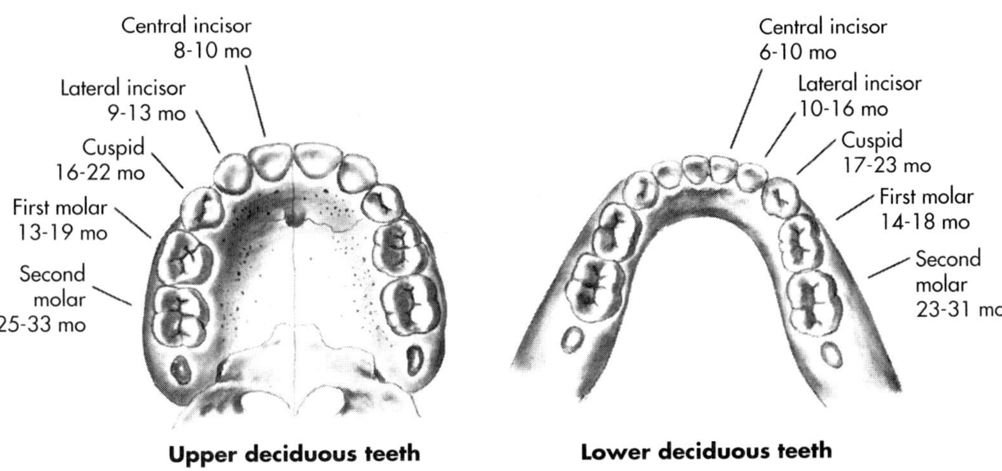

Dentition of deciduous teeth and their sequence of eruption.

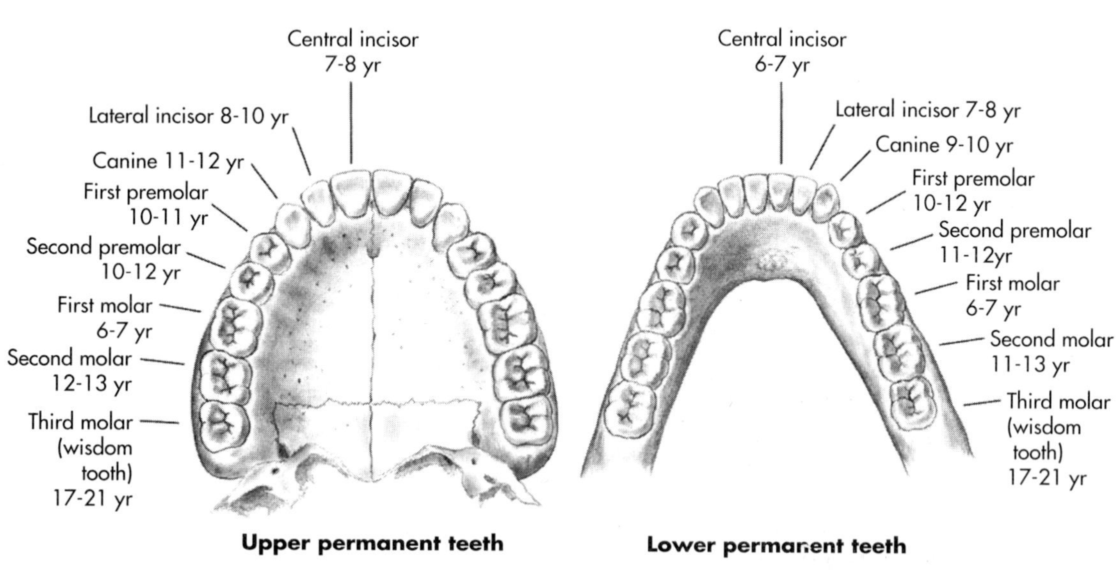

Dentition of permanent teeth and their sequence of eruption.

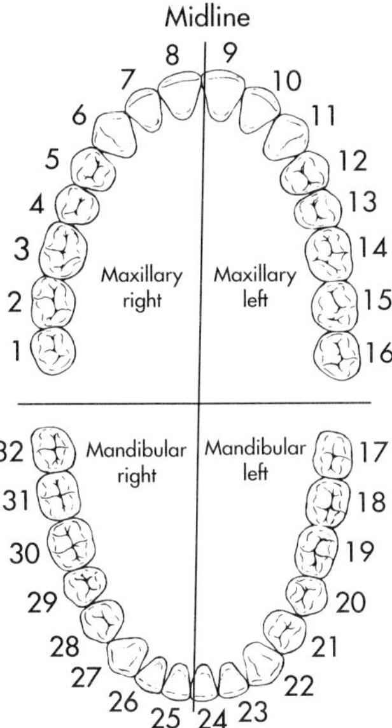

American Dental Association sequential numbering system for permanent teeth. (From Miyasaki-Ching, 1997.)

EAR AND AUDITORY SYSTEM

External Ear

- Inspect both external ears for the following:
  Alignment
  Position
  Shape
  Symmetry
  Skin color
  Uniformity
  Skin intactness
- Inspect the external auditory canal for the following:
  Discharge
  Lesions
- Palpate both external ears and mastoid areas for the following:
  Tenderness
  Swelling
  Nodules

Auditory Canal and Tympanic Membrane

- Inspect the auditory canal for the following:
  Tissue swelling or redness

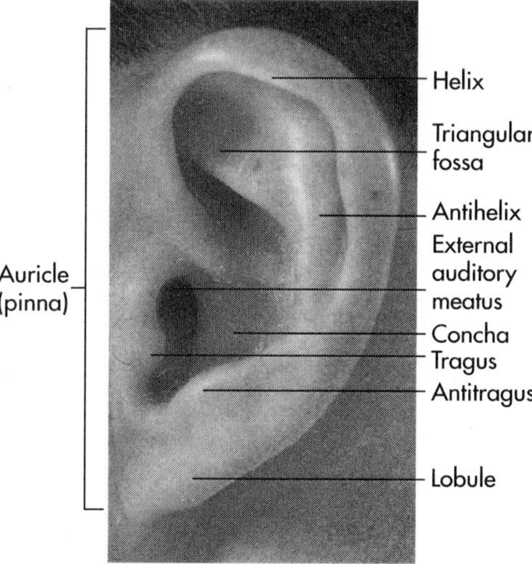

Anatomic structure of the auricle (pinna).

Discharge
Cerumen: amount and characteristics

- Inspect the tympanic membrane for the following:
  Landmarks
  Color
  Contour
  Translucence
  Fluctuation of membrane (if appropriate)

Hearing

- Test the acoustic cranial nerve (VIII) to evaluate auditory function:
  Whispered voice test
  Finger-rubbing test
  Tuning fork tests
  Rine test
  Weber test
- Test the acoustic cranial nerve (VIII) to evaluate vestibular function:
  Romberg test

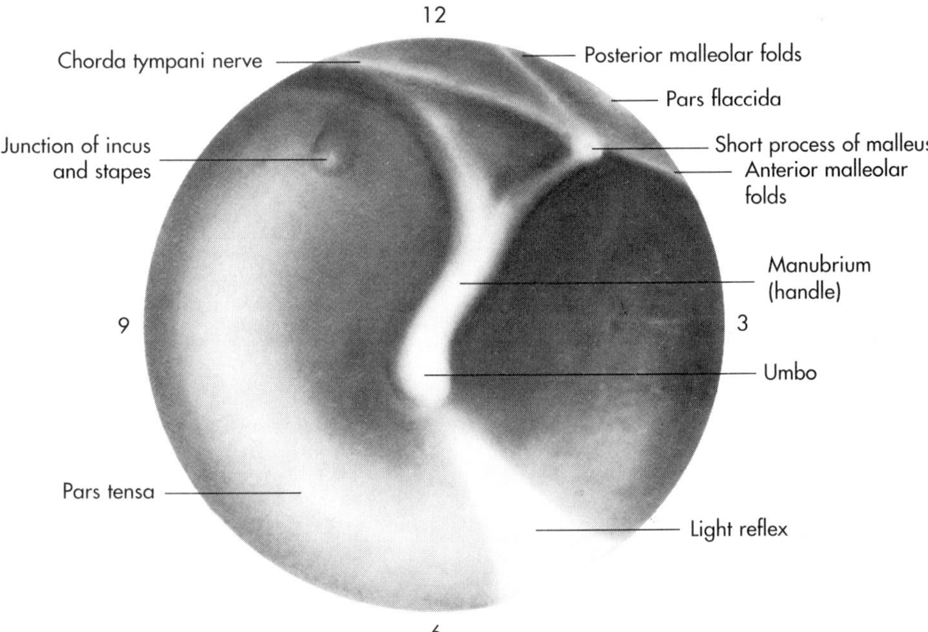

Normal (right) tympanic membrane with usual landmarks noted. (Clock position given as reference.) (Modified from Barkauskus, 1994.)

Noise Levels

DECIBELS (dB)	REPRESENTATIVE SOUND
0	Softest sound normal ear can hear
10	Heartbeat, rustling of leaves
20	Whisper at 1.8 m (5 feet)
30-45	Normal conversation
60	Noise in average restaurant
70-80	Street noises
80	Loud radio at home
90-100	Train
120	Thunder, rock music
140	Jet airplane during takeoff
>140	Pain threshold

From Wong DL: *Nursing care of infants and children,* ed 5, St Louis, 1995, Mosby.

EYES AND VISUAL SYSTEM

Test Visual Acuity

- Test distant vision using the Snellen eye chart or the Snellen E chart.
- Assess near vision using the Jaeger or Rosenbaum card or a newspaper.
- Assess peripheral visual fields using a confrontation test.

Extraocular Muscles

- Inspect the extraocular muscles for movement using the following:
  Six cardinal fields of gaze
  Corneal light reflex
  Cover-uncover test

External Ocular Structures

- Inspect the eyebrows for the following:
  Quality
  Hair distribution
  Underlying skin
  Symmetry

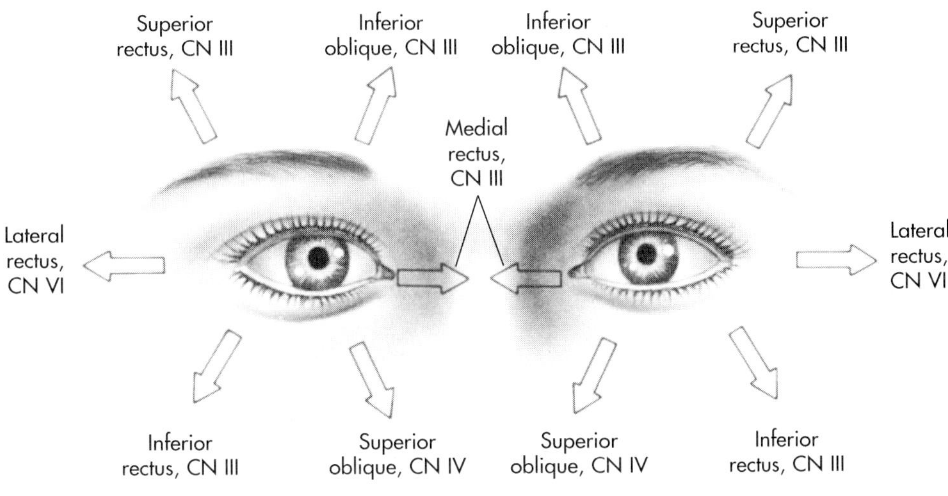

Six cardinal fields of gaze. (From Seidel et al, 1995.)

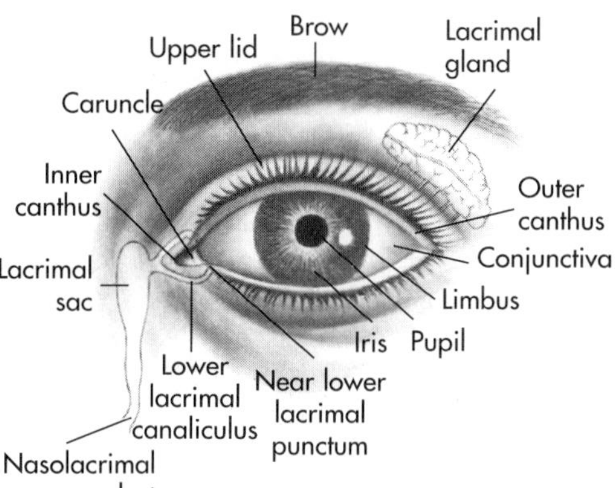

Visible surface of the eye. (From Thompson et al, 1992.)

- Inspect the eyelids and eyelashes for the following:
  Position
  Symmetry
  Closure
  Blinking patterns
  Discharge
  Color
- Inspect and palpate the orbital areas for the following:
  Position
  Indentation
- Inspect the lacrimal puncta for the following:
  Color
  Moisture
  Discharge
  Tenderness
  Nodules

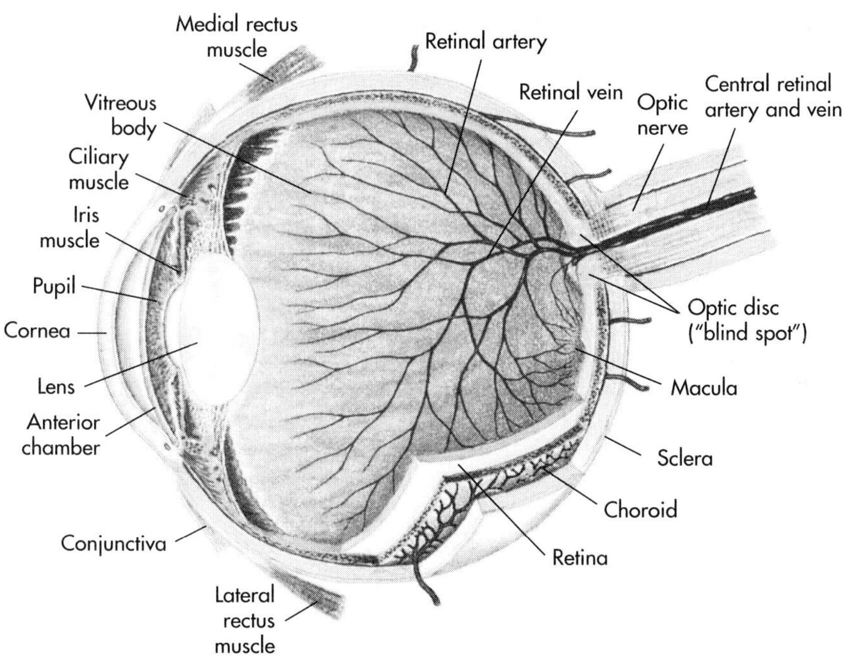

Anatomy of the human eye. (From Seidel et al, 1995.)

- Inspect the conjunctiva and sclera for the following:
  Color and clarity
  Discharge
  Tenderness
  Pterygium
  Crusting
  Lesions
  Nodules
  Foreign bodies
- Inspect the cornea for the following:
  Transparency
  Surface characteristics
- Inspect the anterior chamber for the following:
  Transparency
  Iris surface
  Chamber depth
- Inspect the iris for the following:
  Shape
  Color

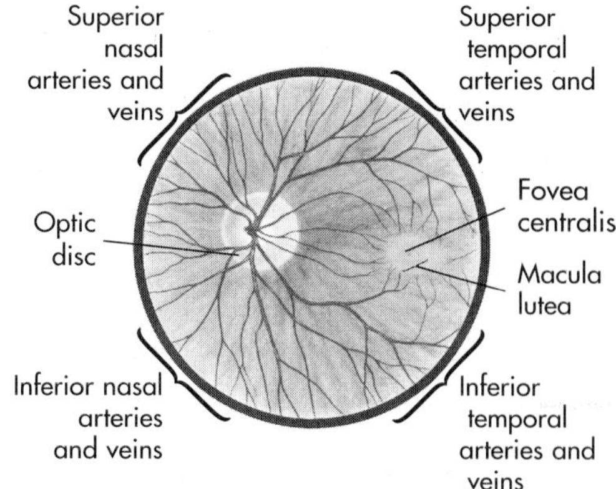

Retinal structures of the left eye. (From Seidel et al, 1995.)

- Inspect the pupils for the following:
  Size
  Shape
  Reaction to light
  Accommodation

Internal Ocular Structures

- Observe the red reflex.
- Inspect the optic disc for the following:
  Margins
  Size and shape
  Color
  Physiologic cup
- Inspect the retinal vessels for the following:
  Color
  Arteriolar light reflex
  Artery-to-vein ratio
  Arteriovenous crossing changes
- Inspect the retinal background for the following:
  Color
  Presence of microaneurysms
  Hemorrhages
  Exudates
- Inspect the macula and fovea centralis for the following:
  Color
  Surface characteristics

LUNGS AND RESPIRATORY SYSTEM

General Presentation

- Inspect the client for the following:
  General appearance
  Posturing
  Breathing effort
  Position of trachea

Chest Wall Configuration

- Inspect the chest wall for the following:
  Form and symmetry
  Muscle development
  Anterior: posterior diameter
  Costal angle

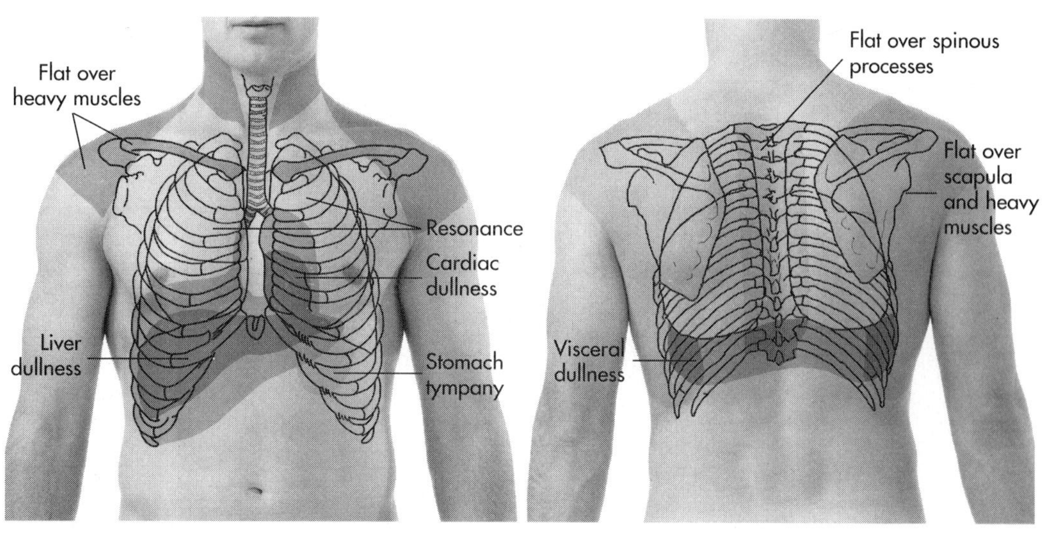

Percussion tones.

General Oxygenation

- Inspect the skin, nails, and lips for color.

Respiratory Rate

- Observe and evaluate the respirations for the following:
  Rate and quality
  Breathing pattern
  Chest expansion

Anterior and Posterior Chest Assessment

- Palpate the trachea for position.
- Palpate the chest wall for the following:
  Symmetry
  Thoracic expansion
  Vocal (tactile) fremitus
- Percuss the thorax for tone and diaphragmatic (respiratory) excursion.
- Auscultate the breath sounds for the following:
  Location of the various sounds
  Presence of adventitious breath sounds
  Vocal sounds (vocal resonance)

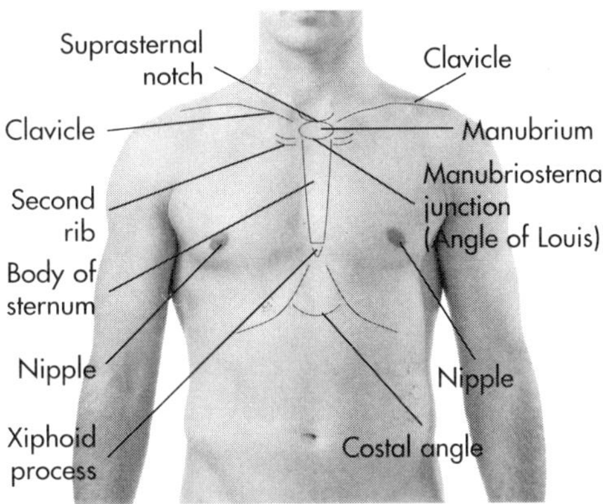

Topographic landmarks of the thorax.

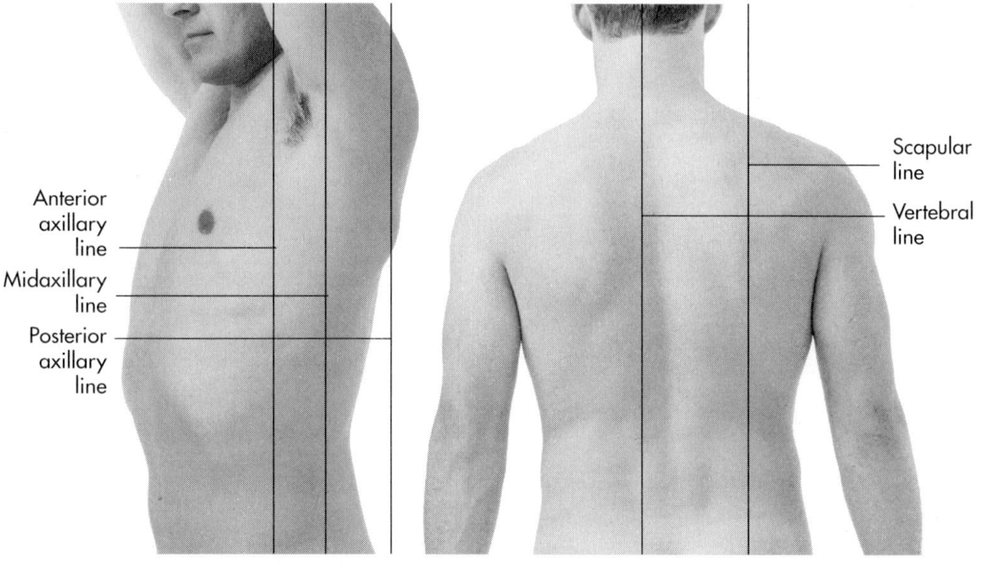

Topographic landmarks of the thorax.—*cont'd.*

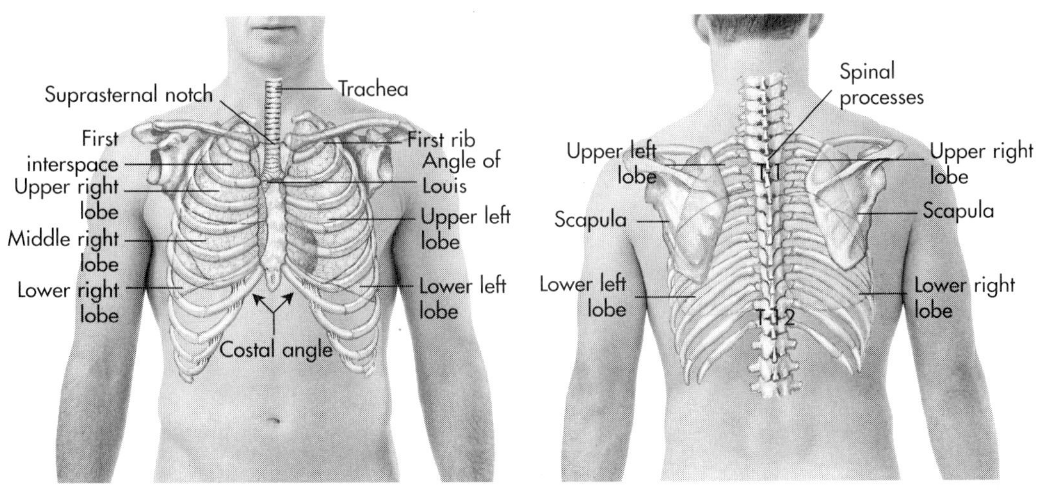

Underlying structures of the thorax.

Characteristics of Adventitious Sounds

Adventitious sounds	Characteristics	Clinical examples
Crackles (previously called rales)		
Fine crackles	Fine, high-pitched crackling and popping noises (discontinuous sound) heard during the end of inspiration. Not cleared by cough.	May be heard in pneumonia, congestive heart failure, chronic bronchitis, asthma, and other restrictive and obstructive diseases.
Medium crackles	Medium-pitched, moist sound heard about halfway through inspiration. Not cleared by cough.	Same as above, but condition is worse.
Coarse Crackles	Low-pitched, bubbling or gurgling sounds that start early in inspiration and extend into the first part of expiration.	Same as above, but condition is worse or in terminally ill clients with diminished gag reflex. Also heard in pulmonary edema and pulmonary fibrosis.

Rhonchi		
Sibilant rhonchi (also called sibilant wheezes) 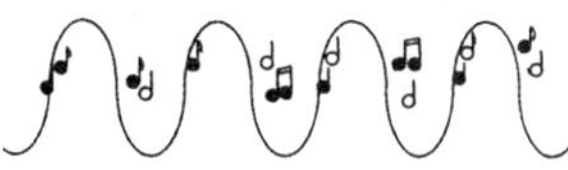	High-pitched, musical sound similar to a squeak. Heard most commonly during expiration, but may also be heard during inspiration. Occurs in small airways.	Heard in obstructive lung diseases such as asthma or emphysema.
Sonorous rhonchi (also called sonorous wheezes) 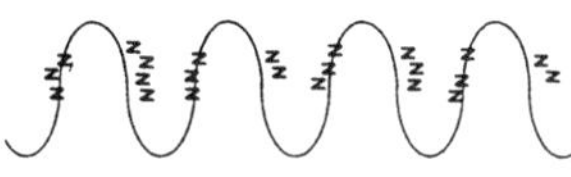	Low-pitched, coarse, loud, low snoring or moaning tone. Actually sounds like snoring. Heard primarily during expiration, but may also be heard during inspiration. Coughing may clear.	Heard in problems causing obstruction of the trachea or bronchus, such as bronchitis.
Pleural Friction Rub 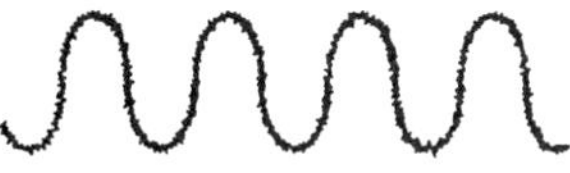	A superficial, low-pitched, coarse rubbing or grating sound. sounds like two surfaces rubbing together. Heard throughout inspiration and expiration. Loudest over the lower anterolateral surface. Not cleared by cough.	Heard in individuals with pleurisy (inflammation of the pleural surfaces).

HEART AND PERIPHERAL VASCULAR SYSTEM

- Evaluate the client's general condition.

Arterial Assessment

Blood pressure

- Palpate, then auscultate arterial blood pressure in both arms.

Pulses

- Palpate each pulse for the following:
  Rate
  Rhythm
  Amplitude
  Contour
- Auscultate the carotid artery for bruits.

Skin, hair, and nails

- Inspect and palpate the extremities for the following:
  Appearance
  Color
  Temperature
  Hair distribution
  Capillary refill

Pulses

Temporal	Radial
Carotid	Femoral
Apical	Popliteal
Brachial	Dorsalis pedis

Pulse Amplitude Ratings

0+	Absent
1+	Diminished, barely palpable
2+	Normal
3+	Full volume
4+	Full volume, bounding hyperkinetic

Venous Assessment

- Inspect the jugular veins for pulsations.
- Estimate jugular venous pressure.
- Inspect and palpate the lower extremities for the following:
  Skin turgor
  Color
  Skin integrity

Cardiac Assessment

- Inspect the anterior chest wall for the following:
  Contour
  Pulsations
  Lifts
  Heaves
  Retractions
- Inspect the apical pulse for visible pulsations.
- Palpate the precordium for the following:
  Pulsations
  Thrills
  Lifts
  Heaves

Calculating Target Heart Rate

The target heart rate (THR) is the recommended rate for increasing cardiorespiratory endurance. To maintain a training effect, a person must sustain activity at his or her THR.

To find a person's target heart rate, subtract the person's age from 220 (the maximum heart rate) and multiply by .60 to .90.

Examples:

For a 20-year-old person (wanting a THR of 80% of maximum)	**For a 40-year-old person (wanting a THR of 65% of maximum)**
Maximum heart rate: 220 − 20 = 200 200 × .80 = 160 THR = 160 beats per minute	Maximum heart rate: 220 − 40 = 180 180 × .65 = 117 THR = 117 beats per minute

- Percuss the heart borders for heart size (optional).
- Auscultate the heart sounds over aortic, pulmonic, tricuspid, mitral, and apical areas for the following:
  Rate
  Rhythm
  Pitch
  Splitting
  Murmurs
  Extra sounds

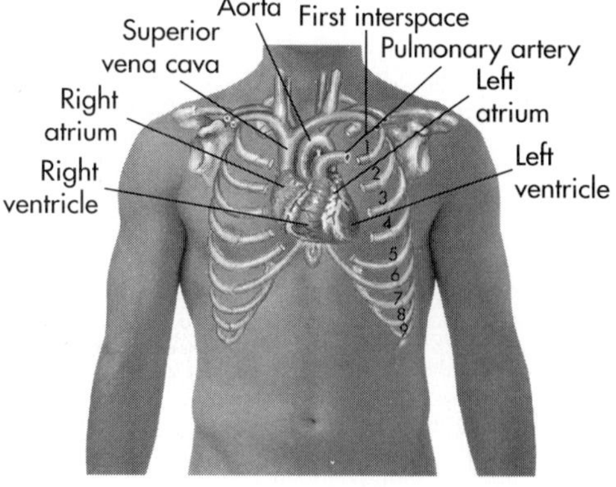

Position of the heart chambers and great vessels.

Pitting Edema Scale

Scale	Degree	Response
1+ Trace	Slight	Rapid
2+ Mild	0-0.6 cm (0-0.25 in)	10-15 s
3+ Moderate	0.6-1.3 cm (0.25-0.5 in)	1-2 min
4+ Severe	1.3-2.5 cm (0.5-1 in)	2-5 min

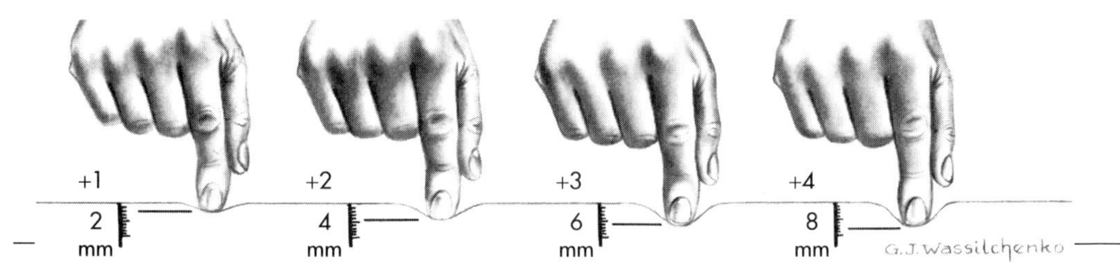

From Canobbio MM: *Cardiovascular disorders,* St Louis, 1990, Mosby.

Technique for Locating Intercostal Spaces for Auscultation of the Heart

A systematic approach is needed for this assessment. Some examiners begin at the apex and proceed upward toward the base of the heart, whereas others begin at the base and proceed downward toward the apex. The sequence is irrelevant as long as the assessment is systematic. Listen first with the diaphragm to hear high-pitched sounds, then with the bell to hear low-pitched sounds.

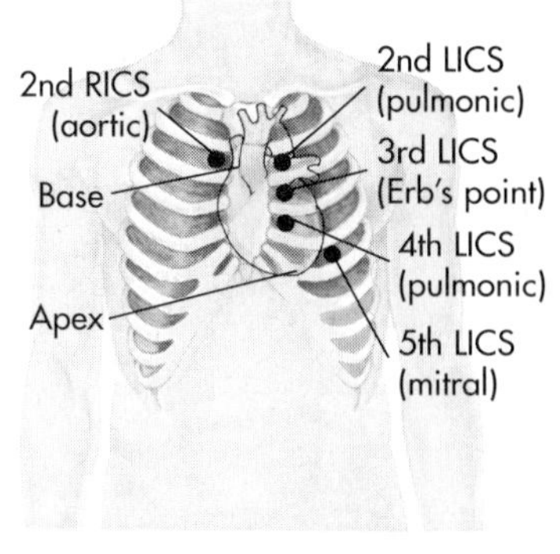

- When auscultating from base to apex, begin at the second intercostal space (ICS). Locate this ICS by palpating the right sternoclavicular joint (where the left clavicle joins the sternum).
- Palpate the first rib, and then move down to palpate the space between the first and second ribs; this is the first ICS.
- Continue palpating downward to the space between the second and third ribs. This is the second ICS at the right sternal border (RSB), the auscultatory site for the aortic valve area. This is not the anatomic site of the aortic valve but the site on the chest wall where sounds produced by the valves are heard best.
- Moving to the left side of the sternum at the second ICS, the area for auscultating the pulmonic valve area is found.
- Remaining at the left sternal border (LSB), move the stethoscope down to the third ICS (Erb's point), an area to which pulmonic or aortic sounds frequently radiate. At the fourth ICS, the LSB is over the tricuspid valve area.
- At the fifth ICS, move the stethoscope laterally to the left midclavicular line where the mitral valve area is located.

BREASTS AND AXILLA

Female

Examination of the breasts and axilla

- Inspect the breasts for the following:
  Size
  Shape
  Symmetry
- Inspect the skin of the breasts for the following:
  Appearance
  Color
  Pigmentation
  Vascularity
  Surface characteristics
- Inspect the areolae for the following:
  Color
  Surface characteristics
- Inspect the nipples for the following:
  Position and symmetry
  Intactness
  Evidence of scaling, lesions, bleeding, or discharge

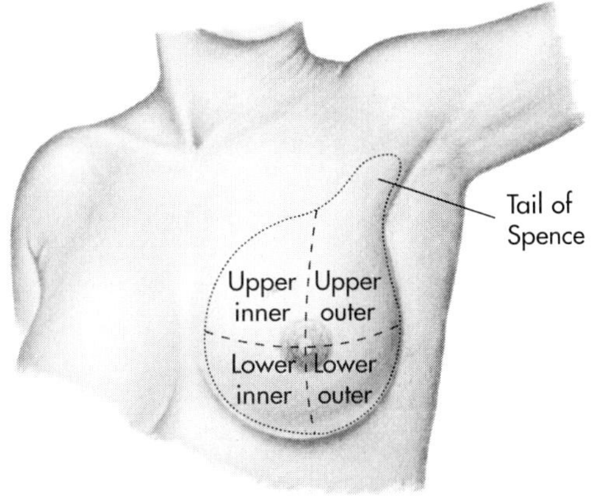

Quadrants of the left breast and axillary tail of Spence. (From Seidel et al, 1995.)

- Inspect the breasts in various positions for the following:
  Bilateral pull
  Symmetry
  Contour
- Inspect the axillae for evidence of rash, lesions, or masses.
- Palpate the breasts and axillae for the following:
  Surface characteristics
  Masses, nodules, tenderness
- Palpate the nipples for the following:
  Surface characteristics
  Discharge
- Teach breast self-examination.

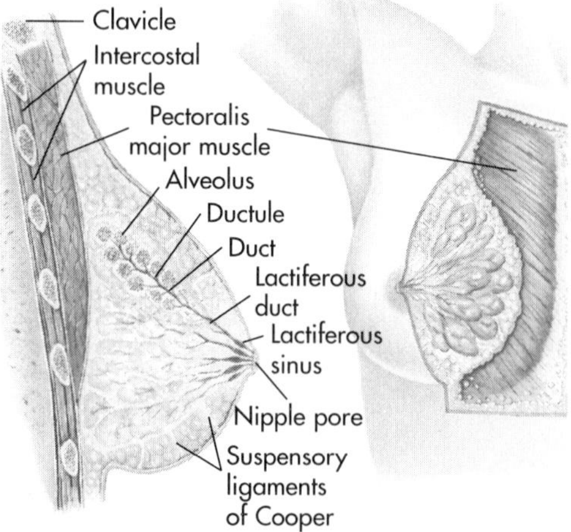

Anatomy of the breast, showing position and major structures. (From Seidel et al, 1995.)

Male

- Inspect the breasts for the following:
  Symmetry
  Color
  Skin lesions
  Enlargement

- Palpate the breasts and areolar areas for the following:
  Tenderness
  Unilateral enlargement
  Masses
- Palpate the nipples for discharge.

ABDOMEN AND GASTROINTESTINAL SYSTEM

Abdomen

- Inspect the abdomen for the following:
  Skin color
  Surface characteristics
  Contour
  Surface movements
- Auscultate the abdomen with the diaphragm of the stethoscope for bowel sounds.
- Auscultate the abdomen with the bell of the stethoscope for the following:
  Arterial (aortic, renal, iliac, femoral) bruits
  Venous hum
- Percuss the abdomen in all quadrants for tones.
- Percuss the liver for span.
- Percuss the spleen for size.
- Percuss the stomach for tympany.
- Palpate the abdomen lightly in all quadrants for the following:
  Tenderness
  Muscle tone
  Surface characteristics
- Palpate the abdomen deeply for the following:
  Tenderness
  Masses
  Aortic pulsation
- Palpate around the umbilicus for the following:
  Bulges
  Nodules
  Umbilical ring
- Palpate the liver for lower border and tenderness.
- Palpate the gallbladder for tenderness.
- Palpate the spleen for the following:
  Border
  Tenderness

- Palpate the kidneys for the following:
  Presence
  Contour
  Tenderness
- Palpate the inguinal nodes for the following:
  Size
  Tenderness
  Mobility
  Contour
- Elicit the abdominal reflexes for presence.

Additional Assessment Techniques for Special Cases

- Percuss the kidneys for costovertebral angle tenderness.
- Assess the abdomen for fluid:
  Shifting dullness
  Fluid wave
- Assess the abdomen for pain:
  Rebound tenderness
  Iliopsoas test
  Obturator test

Anatomic Correlates of the Four Quadrants of the Abdomen

Right Upper Quadrant	**Left Upper Quadrant**
Liver and gallbladder	Left lobe of liver
Pylorus	Spleen
Duodenum	Stomach
Head of pancreas	Body of pancreas
Right adrenal gland	Left adrenal gland
Portion of right kidney	Portion of left kidney
Hepatic flexure of colon	Splenic flexure of colon
Portions of ascending and transverse colon	Portions of transverse and descending colon

Right Lower Quadrant	**Left Lower Quadrant**
Lower pole of right kidney	Lower pole of left kidney
Cecum and appendix	Sigmoid colon
Portion of ascending colon	Portion of descending colon
Bladder (if distended)	Bladder (if distended)
Ovary and salpinx	Ovary and salpinx
Uterus (if enlarged)	Uterus (if distended)
Right spermatic cord	Left spermatic cord
Right ureter	Left ureter

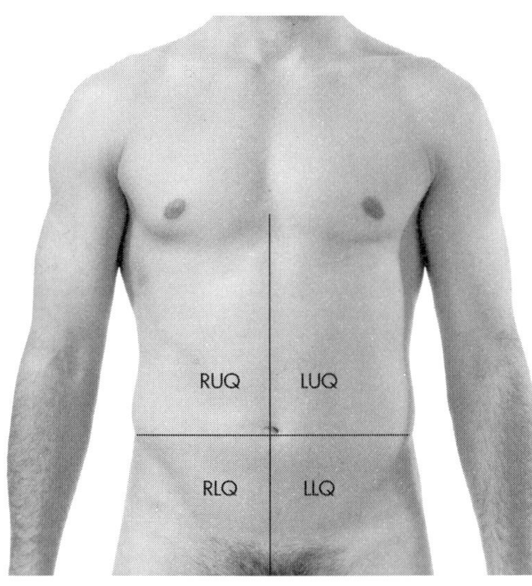

Four quadrants of the abdomen.

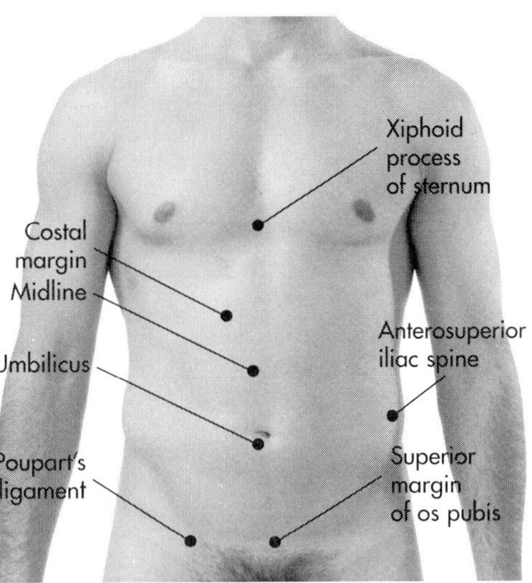

Landmarks of the abdomen.

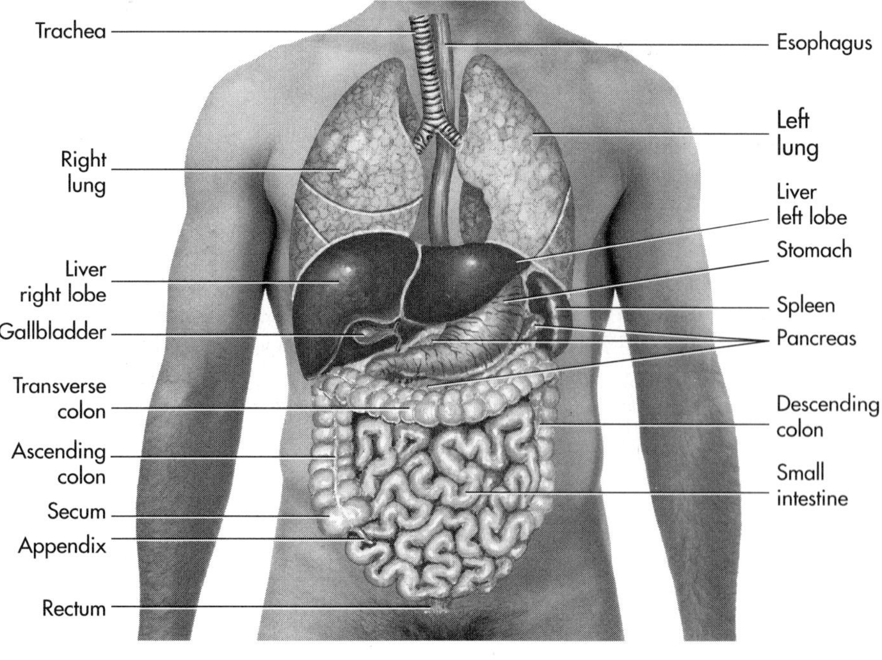

Anatomy of the gastrointestinal system.

- Assess the abdomen for floating mass using the ballottement technique

FEMALE GENITALIA AND REPRODUCTIVE SYSTEM

External Genitalia

- Inspect the pubic hair for distribution.
- Inspect the skin of the mons pubis and inguinal area for surface characteristics.
- Inspect and palpate the labia minora for the following:
  Pigmentation
  Surface characteristics
- Inspect and palpate the labia minora for the following:
  Pigmentation
  Surface characteristics
- Inspect the clitoris for size and length.
- Inspect the urethral meatus, vaginal introitus, perineum, and anus for the following:
  Positioning
  Surface characteristics

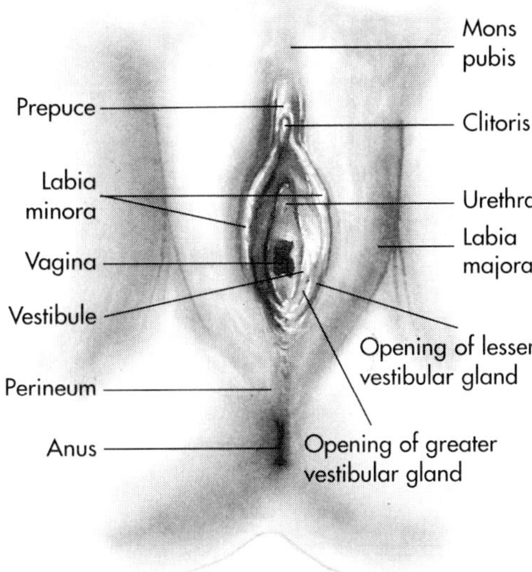

Female external genitalia. (From Seeley, Stephens, and Tate, 1995.)

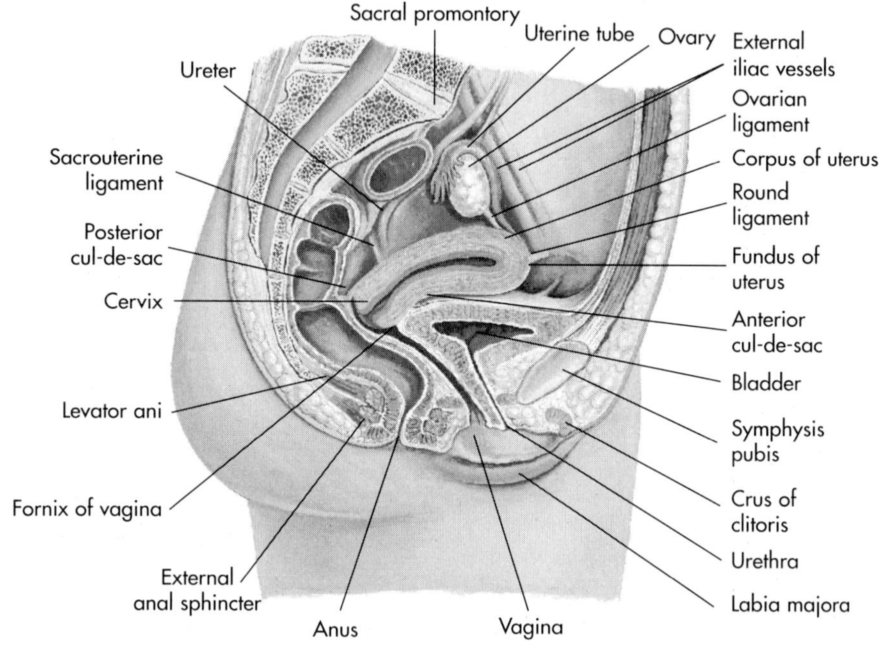

Midsagittal view of female pelvic organs. (From Seidel et al, 1995.)

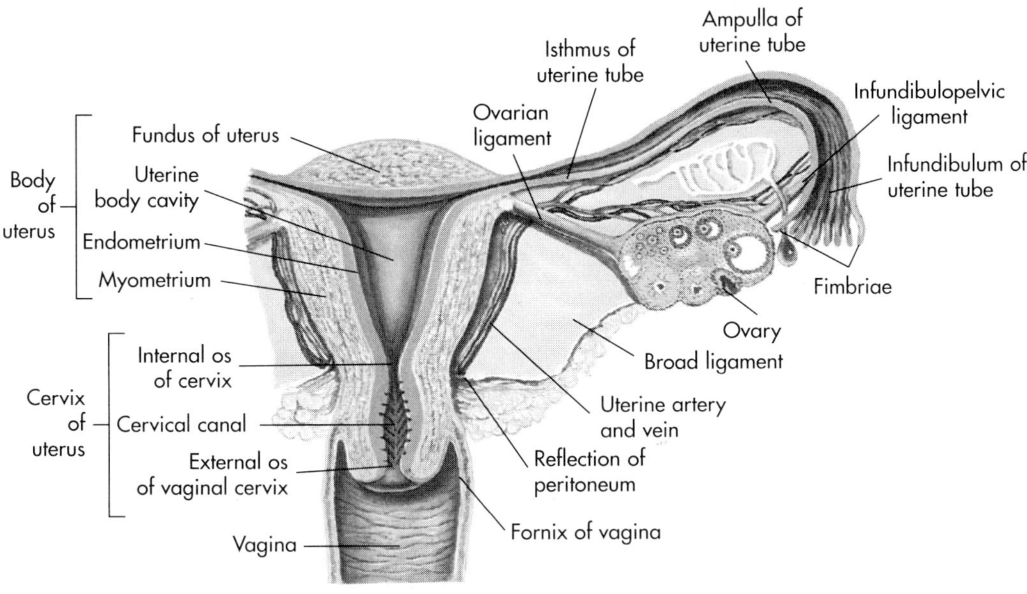

Cross-sectional view of internal female genitalia and pelvic contents. (From Seidel et al, 1995.)

- Palpate the Skene and Bartholin glands for the following:
  Surface characteristics
  Discharge
  Pain of discomfort
- Inspect and palpate muscle tone for the following:
  Vaginal wall tone
  Rectal muscle tone
  Urinary incontinence

Internal Genitalia: Speculum Examination

- Inspect the cervix for the following:
  Color
  Surface characteristics
  Position
  Size and shape
- Inspect the cervical os for discharge.
- Obtain all cervical and vaginal cultures and smears.
- Inspect the vaginal walls for the following:
  Color
  Surface characteristics

Internal Genitalia: Bimanual Examination

- Palpate the vagina, cervix, uterus, and ovaries for the following:
  Position
  Size and shape
  Tissue characteristics
  Mobility
  Pain or discomfort
- Palpate the pelvic region using the rectovaginal examination technique for the following:
  Surface characteristics
  Position of the uterus and adnexa
  Rectal wall characteristics
  Anal sphincter tone

Risk Factors for Cancer

Cervical Cancer
- Onset of intercourse before age of 20 years
- Multiple sex partners
- Infections with human papilloma virus (HPV)
- Cigarette smoking
- Lower socioeconomic status
- Age between 40 and 50 years

Ovarian Cancer
- Age 50 years or older
- Family history of ovarian cancer
- More than 40 years of active ovulation
- Nulliparity or first pregnancy after age 30 years
- High-fat, low-fiber diet; vitamin A–deficient diet
- Prolonged exposure to asbestos and talc

Endometrial Cancer
- Large body frame and obesity
- High-fat diet
- Nulliparity
- Infertility
- Menstrual irregularities
- Late onset of menopause
- Dysfunctional uterine bleeding during menopause
- Adenomatous hyperplasia of the endometrium
- Family history of breast, colon, or ovarian cancer
- History of diabetes or hypertension
- Family history of endocrine cancers

Signs and Symptoms of Sexually Transmitted Diseases (STDs)

There are over 50 STDs. It is impossible to describe the symptoms for all of them. The most common signs and symptoms are the following:

- *Chlamydia* — At first, the woman has no symptoms. When symptoms do appear, usually within 1 to 3 weeks after infection, they include pain on urination, vaginal discharge, or abdominal pain. If left untreated, chlamydia may lead to pelvic inflammatory disease (PID).
- *Genital herpes* — Early symptoms include burning or pain with urination; pain in the buttocks, legs, or genital area; vaginal discharge; or a feeling of pressure in the pelvic area. In a few days, small red bumps appear in the genital area; later the bumps develop into blisters, which open, crust, and then heal. Even after the sores disappear, the herpes virus remains in the body and can reactivate at any time.
- *Gonorrhea* — Often there are no signs. The woman may experience pain or burning when urinating. There may be a yellowish vaginal discharge. Advanced symptoms include bleeding between menstrual periods, swollen joints, fever, or pain in the pelvic area.
- *Genital warts* — These warts are painless, small, bumpy warts that appear on or near the sex organs, usually 3 weeks to 3 months after sex with an infected partner. The warts, which are flesh-colored single or cauliflower-like masses, sometimes develop inside the vagina, on the lips of the vagina, or around the anus.

• *Syphilis*	The first symptom of syphilis, which usually occurs 1 to 12 weeks after sex with an infected partner, often is a painless sore on the genitals. The sore disappears within a few weeks, but the disease progresses. In the second stage, a skin rash appears, along with flulike symptoms. Left untreated, syphilis can lead to blindness, heart disease, brain damage, and even death.
• *Human immunodeficiency virus (HIV) infection and AIDS*	HIV infection and AIDS may produce no symptoms for months or years. As the immune system weakens, the symptoms include swollen lymph glands, fever, night sweats, fatigue, and weight loss.
• *Vaginitis*	The most common symptom is an unusual vaginal discharge. *Trichomoniasis* produces a frothy yellow discharge with a persistent itching or burning and an unpleasant odor. *Yeast infection* produces a discharge that looks like cottage cheese and possibly an intense itch.
• *Gardnerella*	Gardnerella infection causes a grayish-white, watery, strong-smelling discharge.

MALE GENITALIA

Pubic Hair

- Inspect the pubic hair for the following:
  Distribution
  General characteristics

Penis

- Inspect the penis for the following:
  General characteristics
  Color
  Discharge
- Palpate the penis for the following:
  Tenderness
  Induration

Scrotum and Testes

- Inspect the scrotum for the following:
  Texture and general characteristics
  Color
  Asymmetry
- Palpate the scrotum for presence of testes.
- Palpate the testes, epididymides, and vas deferens for the following:
  Location
  Consistency
  Tenderness
  Nodules

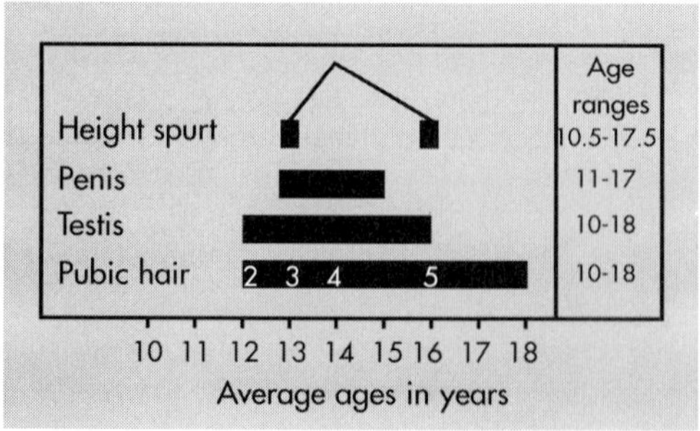

Development of male genitalia and pubic hair. (From Tanner, 1962.)

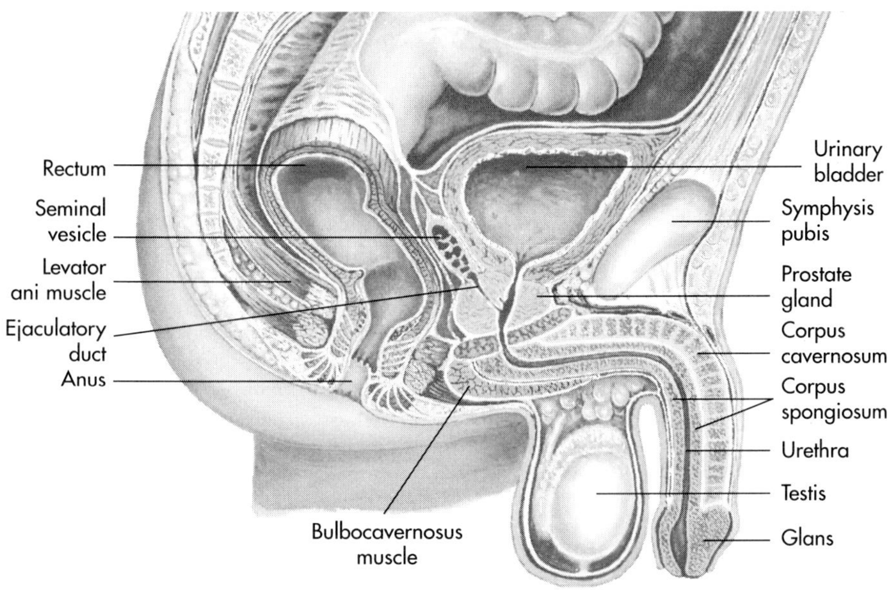

Male pelvic organs. (From Seidel et al, 1995.)

- Transilluminate the scrotum for evidence of the following:
  Fluid
  Masses

Hernia Assessment

- Inspect both inguinal regions for bulges.
- Palpate the inguinal canal for evidence of the following:
  Direct hernia
  Indirect hernia

ANUS, RECTUM, AND PROSTATE

Anus and Rectum

- Inspect the sacrococcygeal and perianal areas for the following:
  Color
  Surface characteristics
  Lesions
  Pilonidal dimpling or tufts of air
- Palpate the coccygeal area for tenderness.
- Inspect the anus for surface characteristics.
- Palpate the anus for sphincter tone.

Prostate Gland

(For male clients)

- Palpate the anterior rectal surface to evaluate the prostate for the following:
  Size
  Contour
  Consistency
  Mobility

Classifications of Prostate Enlargement

Grade	Protrusion into Rectum
Grade I	0.4 to 0.8 in (1 to 2 cm)
Grade II	0.8 to 1.2 in (2 to 3 cm)
Grade III	1.2 to 1.6 in (3 to 4 cm)
Grade IV	Greater than 1.6 in (4 cm)

Stool Evaluation

- Inspect and examine any fecal material for the following:
  Color
  Consistency
  Presence of occult blood by guaiac test

Stool Colors and Significance

Grade	Significance
Bright red	Hemorrhoidal or lower rectal bleeding
Tarry black	Upper intestinal tract bleeding or excessive iron or bismuth ingestion
Light tan or gray	Obstruction of the biliary tract (obstructive jaundice)
Pale yellow	Malabsorption syndrome

MUSCULOSKELETAL SYSTEM

Routine Examination

- Inspect the skeleton and extremities for the following:
  Alignment
  Contour
  Symmetry
  Size
  Gross deformities
- Inspect the skin and subcutaneous tissues for the following:
  Color
  Edema
  Masses
- Inspect the muscles for the following:
  Symmetry
  Size
  Fasciculations
  Spasms

- Observe the gait for the following:
  Conformity
  Symmetry
  Rhythm
- Palpate the bones, joints, and muscles for the following:
  Tenderness
  Heat
  Edema
  Crepitus
- Assess the joints for active and passive range of motion, comparing contralateral sides for the following:
  Tenderness on motion
  Joint stability
  Deformity
  Contracture
- Assess the muscles for strength and compare contralateral sides.

Specific Musculoskeletal Regions

Temporomandibular joint

- Palpate for the following:
  Movement
  Sounds (clicking or popping)
  Tenderness
- Assess muscle strength.

Cervical spine

- Inspect for the following:
  Alignment
  Symmetry
- Palpate for tenderness.
  Masses
  Sensation
- Assess the range of motion of the neck for the following:
  Forward flexion
  Hyperextension
  Lateral bending
  Rotation

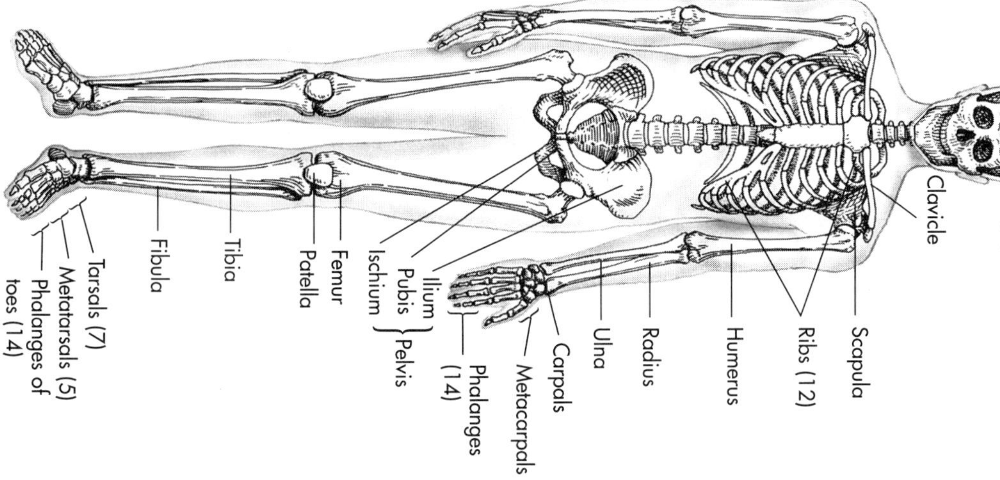

Major bones of the body.
(From Mourad, 1991.)

Skull
Clavicle
Scapula
Ribs (12)
Humerus
Radius
Ulna
Carpals
Metacarpals
Phalanges (14)
Ilium
Pubis
Ischium
Pelvis
Femur
Patella
Tibia
Fibula
Tarsals (7)
Metatarsals (5)
Phalanges of toes (14)

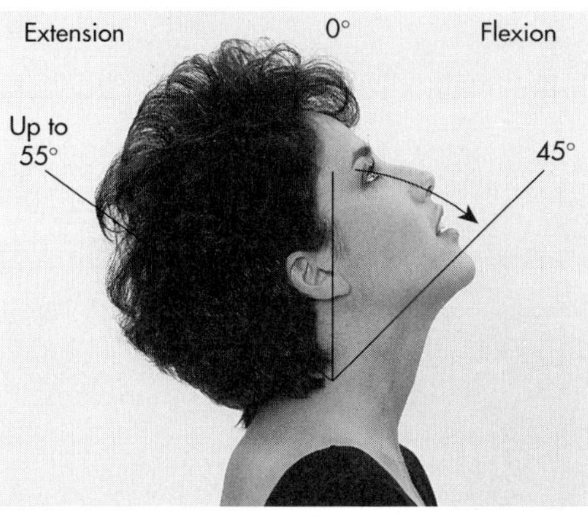

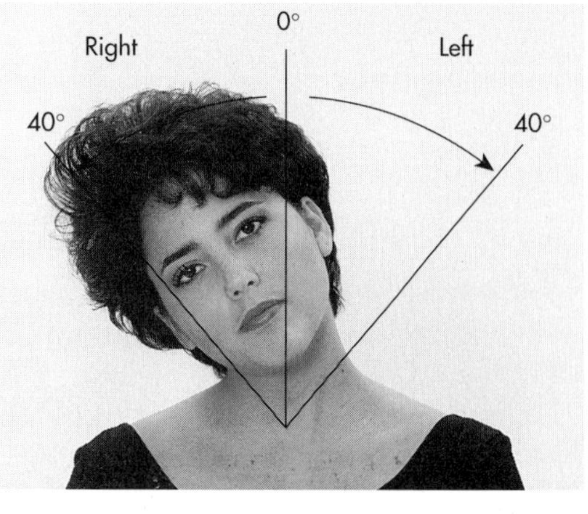

Neck range of motion (ROM).

- Assess the strength of the sternocleidomastoid and trapezius muscles.

Thoracic and lumbar spine

- Inspect the spine, iliac crest, and shoulders for the following:
  Alignment
  Symmetry
- Assess the range of motion for the following:
  Forward flexion
  Hyperextension
  Lateral bending
  Rotation
- Palpate the spinal processes and paravertebral muscles for the following:
  Alignment
  Tenderness
- Percuss the spinal processes for tenderness.

Shoulders

- Inspect the shoulders and shoulder girdle for the following:
  Equality of height
  Contour
- Palpate the shoulders for the following:
  Firmness and fullness
  Tenderness
  Masses
- Assess the strength of the trapezius muscles.
- Assess the range of motion for the following:
  Forward flexion and hyperextension
  Abduction and adduction
  External and internal rotation

Arms

- Assess the muscle strength and compare contralateral sides of triceps and biceps muscles.

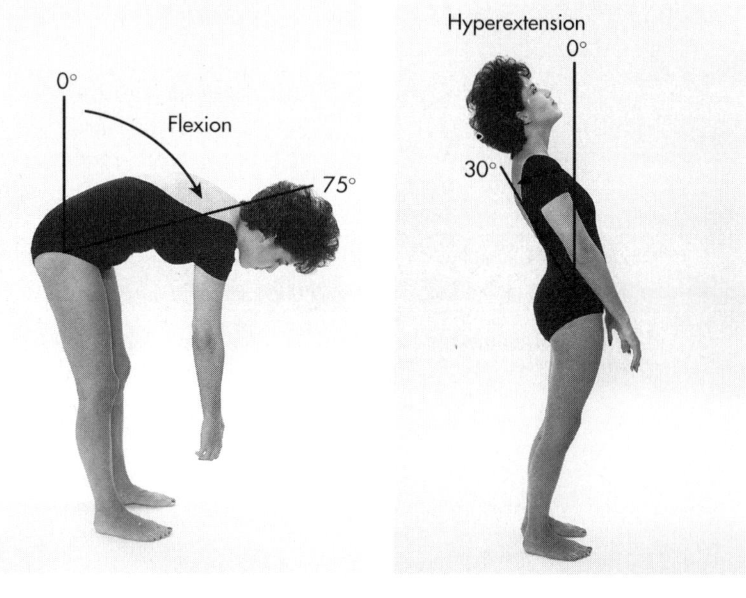

Thoracic and lumbar spine range of motion.

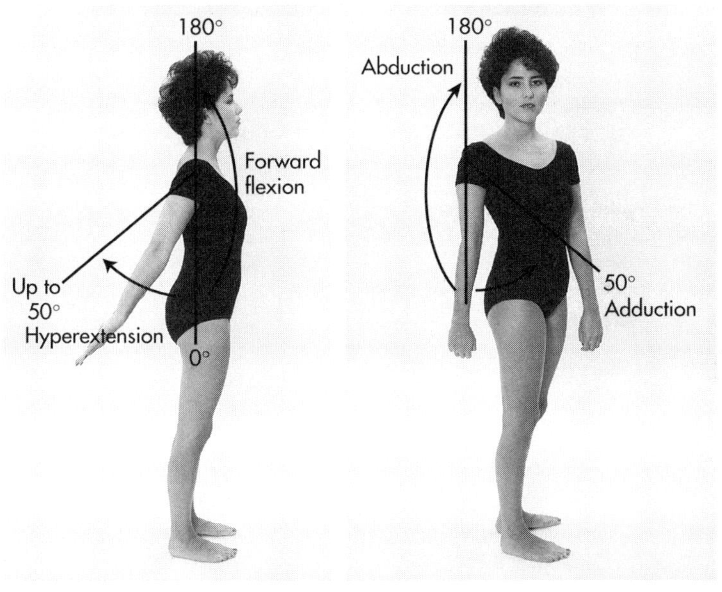

Shoulders range of motion.

Elbows

- Inspect the elbows in flexed and extended positions for the following:
  Contour
  Carrying angle
- Palpate the elbows for tenderness.
- Assess the range of motion for the following:
  Flexion and extension
  Pronation and supination

Hands and Wrists

- Inspect the joints for the following:
  Position
  Contour
  Number of digits
- Palpate each joint for the following:
  Surface characteristics
  Tenderness
- Assess the muscles for strength.
- Assess the range of motion for the following:
  Wrist hyperextension and flexion
  Metacarpophalangeal flexion and hyperextension
  Ulnar and radial motion
  Abduction and adduction of fingers
  Finger flexion (forming fist)
  Thumb opposition

Hips

- Inspect for symmetry.
- Palpate for stability and tenderness.
- Assess the range of motion for the following:
  Flexion and hyperextension
  Internal and external rotation
  Abduction and adduction
- Assess muscle strength.

Knees

- Inspect the knees for the following:
  Alignment
  Edema
  Erythema
- Palpate the knees for the following:
  Contour
  Tenderness

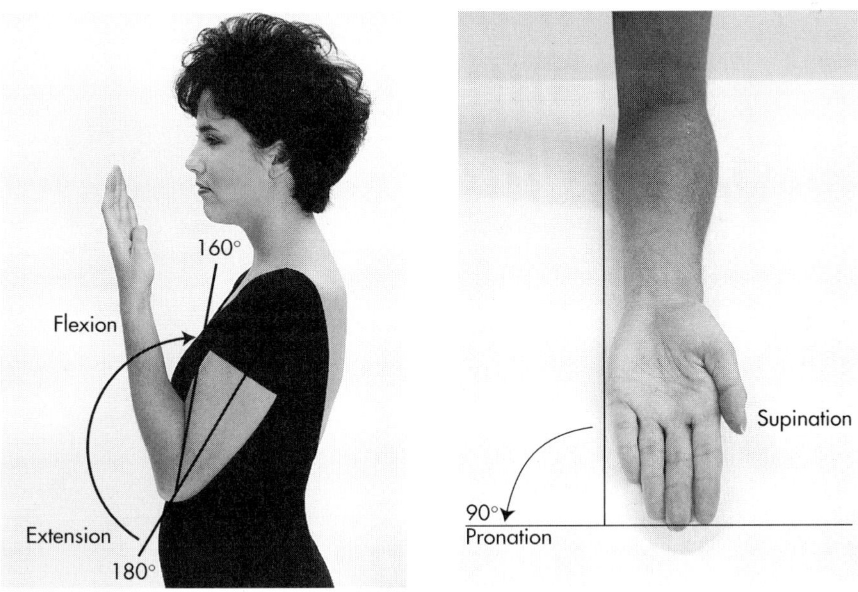

Elbow range of motion.

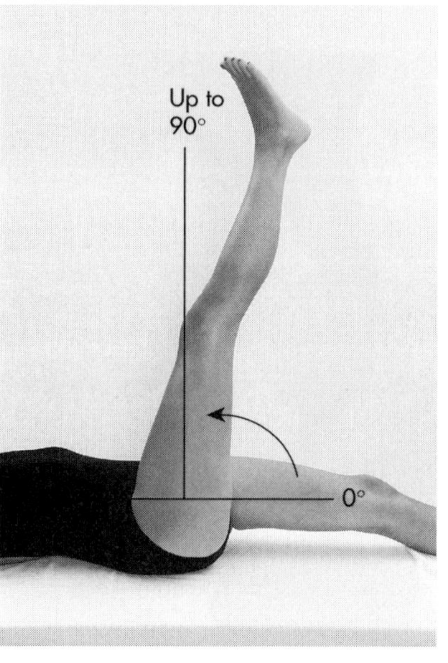

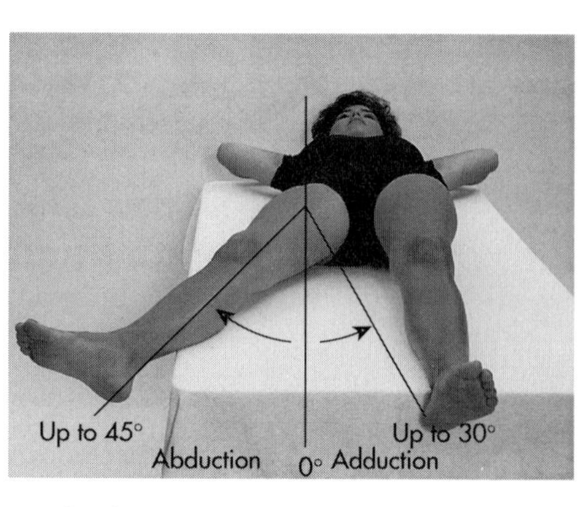

Hip range of motion.

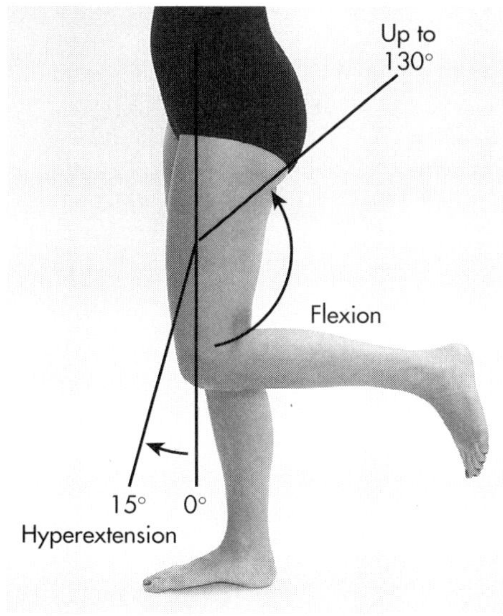

Knee range of motion.

- Assess the range of motion for the following:
  Flexion
  Extension
- Assess muscle strength around the knee.

Feet and Ankles

- Inspect the feet and ankles for the following:
  Contour
  Alignment
  Edema
  Number of toes
- Palpate the feet and ankles for the following:
  Contour
  Tenderness
- Assess the range of motion for the following:
  Dorsiflexion and plantar flexion
  Inversion and eversion
  Abduction and adduction
  Flexion and extension of the toes
- Assess the muscles for strength.

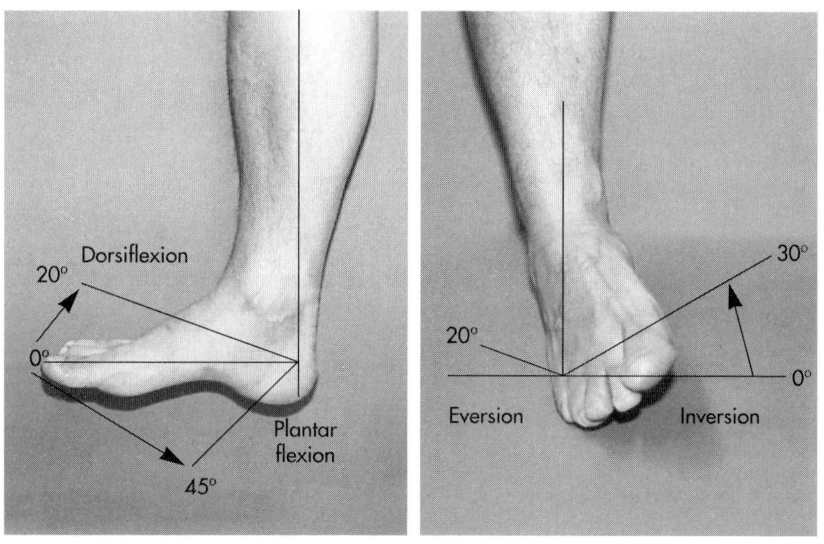

Ankle range of motion.

NEUROLOGIC SYSTEM AND MENTAL STATUS

General Assessment

- Assess the speech for the following:
  Articulation
  Comprehension
  Coherence
  Voice quality
- Assess the nose for smell (olfactory nerve CN I)
- Assess the eyes for the following:
  Visual acuity and peripheral vision (optic nerve CN II)
  Extraocular movement (oculomotor nerve CN III, trochlear nerve CN IV, and abducens nerve CN VI)
  Pupillary constriction and accommodation (oculomotor nerve CN III)
- Assess the face for the following:
  Movement (trigeminal nerve CN V and facial nerve CN VII)
  Sensation (trigeminal nerve CN V)
- Assess the ears for hearing (acoustic nerve CN VIII).
- Assess the mouth for the following:
  Taste (anterior tongue: facial nerve CN VIII; posterior tongue: glossopharyngeal nerve CN IX)
  Gag reflex and movement of soft palate (glossopharyngeal CN IX and vagus nerve CN X)
  Tongue movement, symmetry and strength, and absence of tumors (hypoglossal nerve CN XII)
- Assess the shoulder and neck muscles for the following:
  Strength (spinal accessory CN XI)
  Movement
- Assess cerebellar function for balance and coordination (also tests CN VIII).
- Assess the extremities for the following:
  Muscle strength
  Sensation
  Deep tendon reflexes
- Assess the abdomen for superficial reflexes.

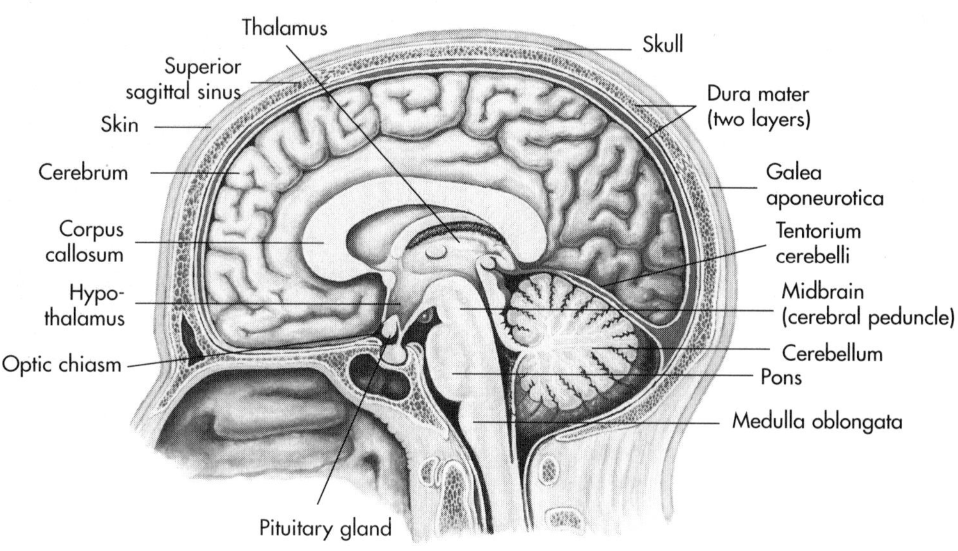

Anatomic structures of the head and brain. (From Chipps and Campbell, 1992.)

- Assess mental status for the following:
  Physical appearance
  Behavior
  Cognitive abilities
  Emotional stability

Scoring Deep Tendon Reflexes

Test the five deep tendon reflexes (triceps, biceps, brachioradial, patellar, and achilles) using a reflex hammer. Compare the reflexes bilaterally. Reflexes are graded on a scale of 0 to 4+, with 2+ being the expected findings. Findings are recorded as follows:

0 = no response
1+ = sluggish or diminished
2+ = active or expected response
3+ = slightly hyperactive, more brisk than normal; not necessarily pathologic
4+ = brisk, hyperactive with intermittent clonus associated with disease

Superficial and Deep Tendon Reflexes

Reflex	Spinal level
Superficial	
Upper abdominal	T7, T8, and T9
Lower abdominal	T10 and T11
Cremasteric	T12, L1, and L2
Plantar	L4, L5, S1, and S2
Deep	
Biceps	C5 and C6
Brachioradial	C5 and C6
Triceps	C6, C7, and C8
Patellar	L2, L3, and L4
Achilles	S1 and S2

From Seidel et al: *Mosby's guide to physical examination,* ed 3, St Louis, 1995, Mosby.

Patient ____________________
Examiner ____________________
Date ____________________

"MINI-MENTAL STATE"

Maximum Score	Score	
		ORIENTATION
5	( )	What is the (year) (season) (date) (day) (month)?
5	( )	Where are we: (state) (county) (town) (hospital)?
		REGISTRATION
3	( )	Name 3 objects: 1 second to say each. Then ask the patient all 3 after you have said them. Give 1 point for each correct answer. Then repeat them until he learns all 3. Count trials and record. Trials
		ATTENTION AND CALCULATION
5	( )	Serial 7s. 1 point for each correct. Stop after 5 answers. Alternatively spell "world" backwards.
		RECALL
3	( )	Ask for the 3 objects repeated above. Give 1 point for each correct.
		LANGUAGE
9	( )	Name a pencil and a watch (2 points) Repeat the following "No ifs, ands, or buts." (1 point) Follow a 3-stage command: "Take a paper in your right hand, fold it in half, and put it on the floor" (3 points) Read and obey the following: CLOSE YOUR EYES (1 point) Write a sentence (1 point) Copy a design (1 point)
	____	Total score
		ASSESS level of consciousness along a continuum ____________________ Alert Drowsy Stupor Coma

INSTRUCTIONS FOR ADMINISTRATION OF MINI-MENTAL STATE EXAMINATION

ORIENTATION

(1) Ask for date. Then ask for parts omitted (e.g., "Can you also tell me what season it is?) 1 point for each correct.

(2) Ask in turn "Can you tell me the name of this hospital?" (town, county, etc.). 1 point for each correct.

REGISTRATION

Ask the patient if you may test his memory. Then say the name of 3 unrelated objects, clearly and slowly, about 1 second for each. After you have said 3, ask him to repeat them. The first repetition determines his score (0-3), but keep saying them until he can repeat all 3, up to 6 trials. If he does not eventually learn all 3, recall cannot be meaningfully tested.

ATTENTION AND CALCULATION

Ask patient to begin with 100 and count backwards by 7. Stop after 5 subtractions (93,86,79,72,65). Score the total correct.

If the patient cannot or will not perform this task, ask him to spell the word "world" backwards. The score is the number of letters in correct order (e.g., dlrow = 5, dlorw = 3).

RECALL

Ask the patient if he can recall the 3 words you previously asked him to remember. Score 0-3.

LANGUAGE

Naming: Show the patient a wrist watch and ask him what it is. Repeat for pencil. Score 0-2.

Repetition: Ask the patient to repeat the sentence after you. Allow only one trial. Score 0 or 1.

3-Stage command: Give patient a piece of blank paper and repeat command. 1 point for each part correctly executed.

Reading: On a blank piece of paper print the sentence "Close your eyes" in letters large enough for the patient to see clearly. Ask him to read it and do what it says. Score 1 point only if he actually closes his eyes.

Writing: Give the patient a blank piece of paper and ask him to write a sentence for you. Do not dictate a sentence; it is to be written spontaneously. It must contain a subject and verb to be sensible. Correct grammar and punctuation are not necessary.

Copying: On a clean piece of paper, draw intersecting pentagons, each side about 1 in, and ask him to copy it exactly as it is. All 10 angles must be present and 2 must intersect to score 1 point. Tremor and rotation are ignored.

Estimate the patient's level of sensorium along a continuum from alert on the left to coma on the right.

"Mini-mental state" test, a standardized screening tool of mental status. The maximum score is 30. Depressed clients without dementia usually score between 24 and 30. A score of 20 or less is found in clients with dementia, delirium, schizophrenia, or an affective disorder. (From Folstein et al, 1985.)

PART THREE

Integrated Physical Examination of Adults

PROCEDURE	BODY PART OR SYSTEMS INVOLVED	CLINICAL STRATEGIES (ADULT AND ELDERLY)
Begin examination with client fully dressed (client may remove shoes for height measurement).		
1. **Assess vital functions and other baseline measurements before asking client to get undressed.**		
Temperature Blood pressure (both arms) Radial pulse Respirations Height Weight Vision testing Snellen chart		If deviation from normal is discovered, reevaluate when associated system is assessed.

Instruct client to undress, put on a gown, and sit on the end of the examination table.

2. **Examine client's hands.**		
Skin surface characteristics	Skin, hair, and nails	Both examiner and client will be at ease if examiner starts with client's hands.
Temperature and moisture of hands		
Characteristics of nails	Heart and peripheral vascular	
Clubbing	Lungs and respiratory	
Skeletal characteristics and/or deformities of fingers and hands	Musculoskeletal	Fine motor neurologic assessment may be included at this point; others find it more convenient to perform neurologic assessment as a clustered procedure toward end of evaluation period.
Range of motion and motor strength of fingers and hands		
Muscle wasting		
Asymmetry		
3. **Examine client's arms from wrists to shoulders.**		
Skin surface characteristics	Skin, hair, and nails	Examine each arm separately.
Muscle wasting	Musculoskeletal	
Asymmetry		May have already been done during vital signs evaluation
Radial pulses: compare one arm with other	Heart and peripheral vascular	Note that, again, neurologic assessment has been delayed.
Range of motion and motor strength of wrists, elbows, forearms, upper arms, shoulders	Musculoskeletal Neurologic	Use make/break techniques.
Palpate epitrochlear lymph nodes.	Lymphatic	

Continued

Procedure	Body part or systems involved	Clinical strategies (adult and elderly)
4. **Examine client's head and neck.**		
Facial characteristics and symmetry	Head and neck	Observe head and neck, gathering as much information as possible.
	Neurologic	
Skin surface characteristics	Skin and hair	Do not touch until after thorough observation.
Symmetry and external characteristics of eyes and ears		
Hair characteristics: texture, distribution, quantity		
Palpate hair and scalp.		Palpate thoroughly; do not be intimidated by hair spray or dirty hair (may need to wash hands before progressing).
Palpate facial bones.	Musculoskeletal	
Client opens and closes mouth for evaluation of temporomandibular joint.		
Client clenches teeth.	Neurologic—CN V (trigeminal nerve)	
Palpate sinus regions.	Paranasal sinuses	
Client clenches eyes tight, wrinkles forehead, smiles,	Neurologic— CN VII, XII (facial, hypoglossal nerves)	Be straightforward; provide client with step-by-step instructions.

sticks out tongue, and puffs out cheeks.		
Eye and near-vision assessment	Eyes and visual	
External eye examination: eyebrows, eyelids, eyelashes, surface characteristics, lacrimal apparatus, corneal surface, anterior chamber, iris		
Near-vision screening and eye function: pupillary response, accommodation, cover-uncover test	Neurologic—CN II, III (optic, oculomotor nerves)	
Extraocular eye movements; vision field testing	Neurologic—CN III, IV, VI, (oculomotor, trochlear, abducens nerves)	Hold chin if head movement occurs.
Internal eye examination: red reflex, disc, cup margins, vessels, retinal surface, vitreous	Eyes and visual	Room must be darkened; should have small amount of secondary light. Instruct client to focus on single object at distance.
Ear and hearing assessment	Ears and auditory	
External ear examination: alignment, surface characteristics, external canal		

Continued

Procedure	Body part or systems involved	Clinical strategies (adult and elderly)
Use whisper test to evaluate hearing.	Neurologic—CN VIII (acoustic nerve)	Room must be quiet.
Otoscopic examination: characteristics of external canal, cerumen, eardrum (landmarks, deformities, inflammation)		Use largest speculum that will fit into canal; if necessary, review technique guidelines for using otoscope.
Rinne and Weber tests	Ears and auditory; neurologic—CN VIII (acoustic nerve)	
Nasal examination: note structure, septum position; use nasal speculum or otoscope to evaluate patency, turbinates, meatus	Nose, paranasal sinuses, mouth, and oropharynx	Even though uncomfortable, should be part of every thorough assessment.
Evaluate sense of smell.	Neurologic—CN I (olfactory nerve)	
Mouth examination: inspect gingivobuccal fornices, buccal mucosa, and gums	Nose, paranasal sinuses, mouth, and oropharynx	
Inspect teeth: number, color, surface characteristics.		If client has dentures, they should be removed.

Inspect and palpate tongue: symmetry, movement, color, surface characteristics.	
Inspect floor of mouth: color, surface characteristics.	
Inspect hard and soft palates: color, surface characteristics.	
Inspect oropharynx: note mouth odor, anterior and posterior pillars, uvula, tonsils, posterior pharynx.	
Palpate tongue and gums.	
Evaluate gag reflex.	Neurologic—CN IX, X (glossopharyngeal, vagus nerves)
Evaluate range of motion of head and neck: instruct client to shrug shoulders against resistance; head movement positions, neck flexion and extension, ear-to-shoulder flexion, chin-to-shoulder rotation.	Musculoskeletal Neurologic—CN XI (accessory nerve)

Continued

Procedure	Body part or systems involved	Clinical strategies (adult and elderly)
Observe symmetry and smoothness of neck and thyroid region.	Head and neck	Client's gown should be lowered slightly so that examiner may fully inspect neck.
Palpate carotid pulses.	Heart and peripheral vascular	
Observe for jugular venous distention.		
Palpate trachea, thyroid (isthmus and lobes), lymph nodes (preauricular, postauricular, occipital, tonsillar, submaxillary, submental, superficial cervical chain, posterior cervical, deep cervical chain, and supraclavicular).	Head and neck; lymphatic	Client may need drink of water to facilitate swallowing during thyroid evaluation.
Auscultate thyroid and carotid for bruits.	Head and neck; heart and peripheral vascular	
Complete assessment of cranial nerves: use cotton swab to evaluate sensitivity of forehead to light touch, cheeks, chin (trigeminal nerve sensory tract)	Neurologic—CN V (trigeminal nerve)	Client should be instructed to close eyes and identify where and when light touch felt.

5. **Asses posterior chest: examiner moves behind client; client seated; gown to waist for men; gown removed but pulled up to cover breasts for women.**		
Observe posterior chest: symmetry of shoulders, muscular development, scapular placement, spine straightness, posture.	Musculoskeletal	
Observe skin: intactness, color, lesions.	Skin	
Observe respiratory movement: excursion quality, depth, and rhythm of respirations.	Lungs and respiratory	
Palpate posterior chest: evaluate muscles and bone structure, palpate excursion of chest expansion; palpate down vertebral column; note straightness.	Musculoskeletal Lungs and respiratory	
Palpate posterior chest for fremitus.		Palpate with pads of fingers while client says "one-two-three."

Continued

Procedure	**Body part or systems involved**	**Clinical strategies (adult and elderly)**
Percuss posterior chest for resonance, respiratory excursion.	Lungs and respiratory	During excursion evaluation, demonstrate to client how to take deep breath and hold it. Measure amount of excursion with ruler.
Percuss with fist along costovertebral angle for kidney tenderness.	Kidney	
Inspect, bilaterally palpate, and percuss along lateral axillary chest walls.	Lungs and respiratory	
Auscultate posterior and lateral chest walls for breath sounds; note quality of sounds heard and presence of adventitious sounds.	Lungs and respiratory	Instruct client to breathe deeply through mouth.
Assess for bronchophony, egophony, and whispered pectoriloquy if adventitious sounds are present.		
6. **Assess anterior chest: move to front of client; client should lower gown to waist.**		

Inspect skin color, intactness, presence of lesions, muscular symmetry, bilaterally similar bone structure.	Skin Musculoskeletal	
Observe chest wall for pulsations or heaving.	Heart and peripheral vascular	
Observe movement during respirations.	Lungs and respiratory	
Observe client's ease with respirations, posture, pursing lips.		
Female breasts: Note size, symmetry, contour, moles or nevi, breast or nipple deviation, dimpling, or lesions; evaluate range of motion of shoulders and regularity of breast tissue during various movements: a. Client's arms extended over head b. Client's arms behind head c. Client' hands behind small of back	Musculoskeletal Breasts and axillae	It is helpful to explain to client basically what she will be expected to do and why before actual examination; may help to alleviate client anxiety as well as facilitate active participation. During examination, it may be helpful to discuss what is being observed; breast self-examination instruction should follow at some point to reiterate these and other aspects of breast examination.

Continued

Procedure	Body part or systems involved	Clinical strategies (adult and elderly)
d. Client's hands pushed tightly against each other at shoulder level e. Client leaning forward slightly so that breasts hang away from chest wall; note symmetry and pull on suspensory ligaments. **Male breasts:** Note size, symmetry, breast enlargement, nipple discharge, or lesions.		
All clients: Palpate lymph nodes associated with lymphatic drainage of breasts; including supraclavicular and infraclavicular, central, lateral, axillary, pectoral, subscapular, scapular, brachial, intermediate, and internal mammary areas.	Lymphatic	

Male clients: Palpate breasts; note swelling or presence of excessive tissue or lumps, nipple discharge, or lesions.		
All clients:		
Auscultate breath sounds of anterior chest from apex to base; note quality, rate, type, presence of adventitious sounds.	Lungs and respiratory	Instruct client to breathe deeply through mouth.
Auscultate heart: aortic area, pulmonic area, Erb's point, tricuspid area, apical area; note rate, rhythm, location, intensity, frequency, timing and splitting of S_1, S_2, S_3, S_4 murmurs.	Heart and peripheral vascular	Examiner must decide whether to start at apical area and work upward or start at aortic area and work downward; examiner should develop routine method of procedure. If examining large-breasted woman, part of auscultatory evaluation may be deferred until client lying down.
All clients:		
Palpate anterior chest wall for stability, crepitations, muscular or skeletal tenderness.	Musculoskeletal	
Palpate precordium for thrills, heaves, pulsations.	Heart and peripheral vascular	Evaluate chest while client is sitting upright and then leaning forward.

Continued

Procedure	Body part or systems involved	Clinical strategies (adult and elderly)
Palpate left chest wall to locate point of maximum impulse (PMI).	Heart	
Palpate chest wall for fremitus, as with posterior chest.	Lungs and respiratory	If examiner has difficulty percussing woman's anterior chest because of large breasts, percuss downward until breast tissue reached; then postpone further percussion until client lies down.
Percuss anterior chest for resonance.		
Female clients:		
Palpate breasts, including all four quadrants, tail of Spence, and areolar area; note firmness, tissue qualities, lumps, areas of thickness, or tenderness.	Breasts and axillae	Client should be comfortably seated with arms resting at side. As before, discuss what is being done so that client can incorporate similar techniques into breast self-examination.
Palpate nipples; note elasticity, tissue characteristics, discharge.	Breasts and axillae	

Assist client to lying or low Fowler position.

7. **Assess anterior chest in recumbent position.**		
Inspect and measure jugular venous pressure for height seen above sternal angle.	Heart and peripheral vascular	Extend footrest for client's legs.
Female breast inspection: Note symmetry, countour, venous pattern, skin color, areolar area (note size, shape, surface characteristics), nipples (note direction, size, shape, color, surface characteristics, possible crusting).	Breasts and axillae	Provide drape for legs and abdomen. Place towel under shoulder of the breast to be evaluated. Instruct client to abduct arm overhead. Explain procedures to client as performed.
Female breast palpation: Note firmness, tissue qualities, lumps, areas of thickness, or tenderness; areolar and nipple area (note elasticity, tissue characteristics, discharge).		After breast palpation, may teach client to palpate own breasts.
All clients:		
Palpate anterior chest wall for cardiac movements or thrills, heaves, pulsations.	Heart and peripheral vascular	

Continued

Procedure	Body part or systems involved	Clinical strategies (adult and elderly)
Auscultate heart: aortic area, pulmonary area, Erb's point, tricuspid area, apical area; note S_1, S_2, S_3, S_4 murmurs (location, rate, rhythm, intensity, frequency, timing, splitting); turn client slightly to left side; repeat assessment of these areas.	Heart and peripheral vascular	
Provide chest drape for females; expose abdomen from pubis to epigastric region.		
8. **Assess abdomen.**		
Observe skin characteristics from pubis to midchest region; note scars, lesions, vascularity, bulges, navel.	Skin and hair	Client should be comfortably positioned with pillow under head and knees slightly flexed to relax abdominal muscles.
Observe abdominal contour.	Abdomen and gastrointestinal	
Observe movement of abdomen, peristalsis, pulsations.	Heart and peripheral vascular Abdomen and gastrointestinal	
Auscultate abdomen (all quadrants); note bowel sounds, bruits, venous hums.	Heart and peripheral vascular	

Percuss abdomen (all quadrants) and epigastric region for tone.	Abdomen and gastrointestinal	
Percuss upper and lower liver borders and estimation of liver span.		Liver percussion should occur at midclavicular line.
Percuss left midaxillary line for splenic dullness.		
Lightly palpate all four quadrants; note tenderness, guarding, masses.		Allow client to become accustomed to examiner's hands.
Deeply palpate all four quadrants; note tenderness, guarding, masses.		Gently but firmly move palpation deeper and deeper until examiner is convinced that abdomen is sufficiently assessed.
Deeply palpate right costal margin for liver border.		Examiner must decide whether to use one-hand or two-hand approach.
Deeply palpate left costal margin for splenic border.		
Deeply palpate abdomen for right and left kidneys.		
Deeply palpate midline epigastric area for aortic pulsation.	Heart and peripheral vascular	Tenderness in epigastic area is normal.
Test abdominal reflexes with pointed instrument.	Neurologic	

Continued

Procedure	Body Part or Systems Involved	Clinical Strategies (Adult and Elderly)
Client raises head to evaluate flexion and strength of abdominal muscles.	Musculoskeletal	Note use of arms or hands to assist; older client may have difficulty with this technique.
Lightly palpate inguinal region for lymph nodes, femoral pulses, and bulges that may be associated with hernia.	Lymphatic Heart and peripheral vascular Abdomen and gastrointestinal	
Client remains lying; abdomen and chest should be draped.		
9. **Assess lower limbs and hips.**		
Inspect client's feet and legs for skin characteristics, vascular sufficiency, pulses; note deformities of toes, feet, nails, ankles, legs.	Skin, hair, and nails Heart and peripheral vascular Musculoskeletal	
Palpate feet and lower legs; note temperature, pulses, tenderness, deformities.	Heart and peripheral vascular Musculoskeletal	
Inspect range of motion and motor strength of toes, feet, ankles, and knees.	Musculoskeletal Neurologic	Motor strength testing may be postponed until patient is seated.

Inspect range of motion and motor strength of hips.		
Palpate hips for stability.	Musculoskeletal	This may be performed last.
Client is lying and adequately draped.		
10. **Assess genitalia, pelvic region, and rectum.**		
Males:		
Inspect and palpate external genitalia, including pubic hair, penis and scrotum, testes, epididymides, and vas deferens.	Genitalia Anus, rectum, and prostate Genitalia and reproductive	If mass in scrotal sac is suspected, transilluminate.
Inspect sacrococcygeal and perianal areas and anus for surface characteristics.		Position client lying on left side with right hip and knee flexed.
Palpate anus, rectum, and prostate gland with gloved finger.		Lubricate gloved finger and slowly insert; wait for sphincter to relax before advancing finger.
Note characteristics of stool when gloved finger is removed.	Anus, rectum, and prostate	

Continued

Procedure	Body part or systems involved	Clinical strategies (adult and elderly)
Females: (client should be lying in lithotomy position):	Genitalia and reproductive Urinary	
Inspect and palpate external genitalia, including pubic hair, labia, clitoris, urethral and vaginal orifices, perineal and perianal area, and anus for surface characteristics.		
Insert vaginal speculum and inspect surface characteristics of vagina and cervix.		
Collect Pap smear culture specimen.		
Perform bimanual palpation to assess form, size, and characteristics of vagina, cervix, uterus, adnexa.		Lubricate first two fingers of gloved hand to be inserted internally; other hand should be positioned on abdomen directly above internal hand.
Perform vaginal-rectal examination to assess rectovaginal septum and pouch, surface characteristics, broad ligament tenderness.		When examination is completed, client should be offered tissue for drying genital area.

Perform rectal examination to assess anal sphincter tone, surface characteristics (anal culture may be obtained).	Anus and rectum	
Note characteristics of stool when gloved finger is removed.		

Client resumes seated position; client should have gown on and have drape across lap.

11. **Assess neurologic system.**		
Observe client moving from lying to sitting position; note use of muscles, ease of movement, and coordination.	Neurologic Musculoskeletal	
Test sensory function by using light and deep (dull and sharp) sensation on forehead, paranasal sinus area, hands, lower arms, feet, lower legs.	Neurologic (sensory function)	Client's eyes should be closed; instruct client to either point to or verbally report area that has been touched. Alternate light, dull, and pin-prick sensations.
Bilaterally test and compare vibratory sensations of ankle, wrist, sternum.		Test bilaterally.
Test two-point discrimination of palms, thighs, back.	Neurologic	Evaluate cortical, discriminatory, and sensory functions.

Continued

Procedure	Body part or systems involved	Clinical strategies (adult and elderly)
Test stereognosis or graphesthesia.		
Test fine-motor functioning and coordination of upper extremities by instructing client to perform at least two of the following: a. Alternating pronation and supination of forearm b. Touching nose with alternating index fingers c. Rapidly alternating finger movements to thumb d. Rapidly moving index finger between nose and examiner's finger	Neurologic	Perform technique bilaterally and compare responses (evaluates the proprioception and cerebellar function).
Test and bilaterally compare fine-motor functioning and coordination of lower extremities by instructing client to run heel down tibia of opposite leg.		

Alternately cross legs over knee.	Musculoskeletal	
Test proprioception by moving the toe up and down.	Neurologic	If client shows any neurologic problems, evaluate by Babinski and ankle clonus tests (evaluates the client's reflex status).
Test and bilaterally compare deep tendon reflexes, including the following: a. Biceps tendon b. Triceps tendon c. Brachioradialis tendon d. Patellar tendon e. Achilles tendon		
Instruct client to stand.		
12. **Palpate scrotum and inguinal region (male).**	Genitalia	
Palpate scrotum and inguinal region for characteristics and hernias.	Genitalia	Instruct client to bear down or cough during hernia evaluation.

Continued

Procedure	Body part or systems involved	Clinical strategies (adult and elderly)
13. **Assess neurologic and musculoskeletal system.**		
Assess client's gait: observe and palpate straightness of client's spine as client stands and bends forward to touch toes.	Musculoskeletal Neurologic	Elderly clients may not be able to do this. Client's age and general ability may help define which technique to use.
With client's waist stabilized, evaluate hyperextension, lateral bending, rotation of upper trunk.	Musculoskeletal	
Assess proprioception and cerebellar and motor functions by using at least two of the following: a. Romberg test (eyes closed) b. Walking straight heel-to-toe formation c. Standing on one foot and then other (eyes closed) d. Hopping in place on one foot and then other e. Knee bends	Neurologic	Protect client from falling by remaining close and ready to catch him or her if necessary. Elderly clients may not be able to do this.

PART FOUR

Integrated Physical Examination of Infants and Children

Age and preparation	Assessment procedures	Body part or system involved
Newborn to 6 months: infant undressed, lying on examination table	Obtain history, highlighting developmental or problem areas.	
	Check vital signs: temperature, pulse, respiration.	
	Record weight, length, chest, and head circumference.	
	Observe child lying on examination table; note color, general health, body symmetry, gross motor movement, alertness, gross and fine motor development, language development, social adaptive development,	Heart and peripheral vascular, neurologic, musculoskeletal, skin, eyes and visual, ears and auditory

Continued

Age and Preparation	Assessment Procedures	Body Part or System Involved
	skin characteristics, and response to sound and vision stimulation.	
	Examine and manipulate hands, arms, shoulders, feet, legs; note range of motion and tone.	Musculoskeletal, neurologic
	Examine skin over extremities, chest, abdomen, and back.	Skin and hair
	Auscultate thorax, lungs, heart, abdomen.	Lungs and respiratory, heart and peripheral vascular, abdomen and gastrointestinal
	Palpate and examine external characteristics of head, neck, face, axillary region.	Lymphatic, head and neck, eyes and visual, ears and auditory, nose, mouth, oropharynx
	Palpate thorax, abdomen, and umbilical area.	Lungs and respiratory, abdomen and gastrointestinal
	Observe and palpate external genitalia, inguinal area, hip stability.	Genitalia, musculoskeletal
	Examine eyes with ophthalmoscope.	Eyes and visual
	Examine mouth, teeth (development), tongue, posterior pharynx, nose.	Nose, mouth, and oropharynx
	Examine ears with otoscope.	Ears and auditory

6 months to 2 years: child in diaper, sitting on parent's lap; examiner's chair should be in front of parent's chair, and examiner's knees should touch parent's; during supine examination, child may lie on parent's or examiner's lap	Obtain history highlighting developmental or problem areas.	
	Perform developmental, social, vision, speech, hearing, and fine and gross motor assessment during play and initial "get acquainted" period.	Neurologic, eyes and visual, speech, ears and auditory, musculoskeletal
	Record weight, length, and chest and head circumferences (until 18 months of age).	
	Check vital signs, including blood pressure in children over 18 months of age (may be postponed until later if child becomes agitated).	
	Auscultate lungs and heart.	Lungs and respiratory, heart and peripheral vascular
	Examine skin over extremities, chest, abdomen, and back.	Skin and hair
	Examine and manipulate hands, arms, shoulders, feet, legs; note range of motion and tone.	Neurologic, musculoskeletal

Continued

Age and Preparation	Assessment Procedures	Body Part or System Involved
	Palpate and examine external characteristics of head, neck, face, axillary region.	Lymphatic, head and neck, eyes and visual, ears and auditory, nose, mouth, oropharynx
	Auscultate abdomen with child in supine position on parent's or examiner's lap.	Abdomen and gastrointestinal
	Palpate thorax, abdomen, and umbilical area.	Lungs and respiratory, abdomen
	Observe and palpate external genitalia, inguinal area, and hip stability.	Genitalia, musculoskeletal
	Examine eyes with ophthalmoscope.	Eyes and visual
	Examine mouth, teeth (development), tongue, posterior pharynx, nose.	Nose, mouth, nasopharynx, head and neck
	Examine ears with otoscope.	Ears, auditory

2 to 4 years: child undressed to underpants; may be examined either on parent's lap or examination table; much of assessment may be informal as examiner observes and plays with child	Same assessment procedures as for child age 6 months to 2 years.
4 to 6 years: child undressed to underpants, sitting on examination table; assessment should move toward adult format; child's developmental immaturity may necessitate that examiner alter various examination techniques to facilitate child's participation and correct response	Same assessment procedures as for child age 6 months to 2 years
Over 6 years old: child in gown on examination table	Same assessment procedures and approach as for adult client

Expected Development of Infants

Age	Fine motor	Gross motor	Social/adaptive	Language
1 month	Follows with eyes to midline Hands predominantly closed Strong grasp reflex	Turns head to side Keeps knees tucked under abdomen When pulled to sitting position, has gross head lag and rounded, swayed back	Regards face	Responds to bell Cries in response to displeasure Makes sounds during feeding
2 months	Follows objects well; may not follow past midline Hands frequently open	Holds head in same plane as rest of body Can raise head and maintain position; looks downward	Smiles responsively	Vocalizes (not crying) Cries become differentiated Coos
3 months	Follows past midline When in supine position puts hands together; will hold hands in front of face Pulls at blanket and clothes	Raises head to 45° angle Maintains posture Looks around with head May turn from prone to side position	Shows interest in surroundings	Laughs Coos, babbles, chuckles

		When pulled into sitting position, shows only slight head lag	Becomes bored when left alone	
4 months	Grasps rattle Plays with hands together Inspects hands Carries objects to mouth	Actively lifts head up and looks around Will roll from prone to supine position When pulled to sitting position, no longer has head lag When held in standing position, attempts to maintain some weight support	Begins to show memory	Squeals Vocalizations change with mood
5 months	Can reach and pick up object May play with toes	Able to push up from prone position and maintain weight on forearms Rolls from prone to supine and back to prone Maintains straight back when in sitting position	Smiles spontaneously Playful, with rapid mood changes Distinguishes family	Uses vowel-like cooing sounds with consonantal sounds (e.g., *ah-goo*)

Continued

Expected Development of Infants—*Cont.*

Age	Fine motor	Gross motor	Social/adaptive	Language
6 months	Will hold spoon or rattle Will drop object and reach for second offered object Holds bottle	Begins to raise abdomen off table Sits, but posture still shaky May sit with legs apart; holds arms straight as prop between legs Supports almost full weight when pulled to standing position	Recognizes parents Holds out arms to be picked up	Begins to imitate sounds Uses one-syllable sounds (e.g., *ma, mu, da, di*)
7 months	Can transfer object from one hand to other Grasps objects in each hand Bangs cube on table	Sits alone; still uses hands for support When held in standing position, bounces Puts feet to mouth	Fearful of strangers Plays peek-a-boo Keeps lips closed when dislikes food	Says four distinct vowel sounds "Talks" when others are talking
8 months	Beginning thumb-finger grasping Releases object at will	Sits securely without support Bears weight on legs when supported	Responds to word "no" Dislikes diaper changes	Makes consonant sounds *t, d, w* Uses two syllables such as *dada,* but

	Grasps for toys out of reach	May stand holding on		does not ascribe meaning to them
9 months	Continued development of thumb-finger grasp May bang objects together Use of dominant hand evident	Steady sitting; can lean forward and still maintain position Begins creeping (abdomen off floor) Can stand holding onto established object when placed in that position	Seems interested in pleasing parent Show fears of going to bed and being left alone	Responds to simple commands Comprehends *no-no*
10 months	Practices picking up small objects Points with one finger Will offer toys to people but unable to let go of objects	Can pull self into standing position; unable to let self down again Stands while holding on to furniture	Inhibits behavior in response to command *no-no* Repeats actions that attract attention Plays interactive games such as pat-a-cake Cries when scolded	Says *da da, ma ma* with meaning Comprehends *bye-bye*
11 months	Holds crayon to mark on paper	Moves about room holding onto objects	Experiences satisfaction when task is accomplished	Imitates speech sounds

Continued

Expected Development of Infants—*Cont.*

Age	Fine Motor	Gross Motor	Social/Adaptive	Language
	Drops object deliberately for it to be picked up	Preparing to walk independently; wide-base stance Stands securely holding on with one hand	Reacts to restrictions with frustration Rolls a ball to another upon request	
12 months (1 year)	May hold cup and spoon and feed self fairly well with practice Can offer toys and release them Releases cube in cup	Able to twist and turn and maintain posture Able to sit from standing position May stand alone, at least momentarily	Shows emotions of jealousy, affection, anger, fear May develop habit of "security blanket" or favorite toy	*Da da* or *ma ma* specific Recognizes objects by name Imitates animal sounds Understands simple verbal commands (e.g., "*Give it to me*")

Expected Development of Toddlers

Age	Fine motor	Gross motor	Social/adaptive	Language
15 months	Can put raisins into bottle Will take off shoes and pull toys Builds tower of 2 cubes Scribbles spontaneously Uses cup well, but rotates spoon	Walks alone well Able to seat self in chair Creeps up stairs Cannot throw ball without falling	Tolerates some separation from parents Begins to imitate parents' activities (e.g., sweeping, mowing lawn)	Says 10 or more words "Asks" for objects by pointing Uses *no* even when agreeing with request
18 months	Builds tower of 3 to 4 cubes Turns pages in book 2 or 3 at a time Manages spoon without rotating	May walk up and down stairs holding hand May show running ability	Imitates housework Temper tantrums may be more evident Has beginning awareness of ownership (e.g., *my toy*)	Says 10 or more words Points to 2 or 3 body parts
24 months (2 years)	Able to turn doorknob Able to take off shoes and socks Able to build 7- to 8-block tower	May walk up stairs by self, two feet on each step Able to walk backward Able to kick ball	Parallel play demonstrated Pulls people to show them something Increased independence from mother	Has vocabulary of 300 words Uses 2- or 3-word phrases Uses pronouns *I, you* Uses first name

Continued

Expected Development of Toddlers—*Cont.*

Age	Fine motor	Gross motor	Social/adaptive	Language
	Dumps raisins from bottle following demonstration Turns pages in book one at a time			Refers to self by name
30 months (2½ years)	Able to build 8-block tower Scribbling techniques continue Feeding self with increased neatness Dumps raisins from bottle spontaneously	Able to jump from object Walking becomes more stable; wide-base gait decreases Throws ball overhanded	Separates easily from mother In play, helps put things away In toileting, only needs help to wipe Begins to notice sex differences	Gives first and last names Uses plurals Refers to self by appropriate pronoun Names one color

Expected Development of Preschoolers

Age	Fine motor	Gross motor	Social/adaptive	Language
36 months (3 years)	Can unbutton front buttons Copies vertical lines within 30° Copies zero Begins to use fork	Walks up stairs, alternating feet on steps Walks down stairs, two feet on each step Pedals tricycle Jumps in place Able to perform broad jump	Dresses self with help with back buttons Pulls on shoes Parallel play Able to share toys	Vocabulary of 900 words Uses complete sentences Constantly asks questions
48 months (4 years)	Able to copy plus sign (+) Picks longer line 3 out of 3 times Uses scissors Can lace shoes	Walks down stairs, alternating feet on steps Able to button large front buttons Able to balance on one foot for approximately 5 seconds Catches ball	Play is associative Imaginary friend is common Boasts and tattles Selfish, impatient, rebellious	Gives first and last names Has 1500-word vocabulary Uses words without knowing meaning Questioning is at a peak

Continued

Expected Development of Preschoolers—*Cont.*

Age	Fine Motor	Gross Motor	Social/Adaptive	Language
60 months (5 years)	Able to dress self with minimal assistance Able to draw 3-part human figure Draws square (■) following demonstration Colors within lines	Hops on one foot Catches ball bounced to him or her two out of three times Able to demonstrate heel-toe walking Jumps rope	Eager to follow rules Less rebellious Relies on outside authority to control the world	Has 2100-word vocabulary Recognizes 3 colors Asks meanings of words Uses sentences of 6 to 8 words

PART FIVE

Documentation Format

SUBJECTIVE DATABASE (HISTORY)

- **Biographic data**
- **Reason for visit**
- **Present health status**
- **Current health data**
  Immunizations
  Allergies
  Last examination
- **Past health status**
  Childhood illnesses
  Serious or chronic illnesses
  Serious accidents or injuries
  Hospitalizations
  Surgeries
  Emotional health
  Obstetric health
- **Family history**
- **Review of physiologic systems**
  General
  Nutritional
  Integumentary
  Head and neck
  Eyes
  Ears, nose, and mouth
  Breasts
  Cardiovascular

Respiratory
Hematolymphatic
Gastrointestinal
Urinary
Genital
Musculoskeletal
Central nervous system
Endocrine
Allergic and immunologic responses

- **Psychosocial history**

General status
Response to illness
Significant others
Occupational history
Educational level
Activities of daily living
Habits
Financial status

- **Health maintenance efforts**

Maintenance of self-health
Health care patterns

- **Environmental health**

General assessment
Employment
Home
Neighborhood
Community

OBJECTIVE DATABASE (PHYSICAL EXAMINATION)

- **Vital statistics**

Age
Race
Nutritional status
Height
Weight
Temperature
Pulse
Blood pressure (both arms, lying and sitting)
Communication skills

- **General statement of appearance**
- **Integumentary system (skin, hair, and nails)**

Color
Integrity

Texture
Presence or absence of lesions, edema, unusual odors
Distribution and texture of hair

- **Head and neck**
  Size, symmetry, and contour of head and face
  Edema or puffiness
  Palpation of lymph nodes
  Palpation of thyroid
  Palpation of sinuses
- **Nose**
  Position, including septum
  Nasal patency
  Presence of polyp(s)
  Appearance of turbinates
- **Mouth and pharynx**
  Condition and alignment of teeth
  Color and characteristics of tongue, mucosa, pharynx, gums
  Position and appearance of tonsils and palate
  Symmetry and movement of tongue and uvula
  Taste and gag reflex
- **Ears and auditory system**
  Position and alignment of auricles
  Surface characteristics of external ear and canal
  Characteristics of temporomandibular joint
  Rinne and Weber test
- **Eyes and visual systems**
  Visual acuity and visual fields
  Surface characteristics of eyes
  Extraocular movements
  Corneal light reflex
  Characteristics of cornea
  Consensual response to light
  Findings from ophthalmoscopic examination
- **Lungs and respiratory system**
  Chest wall configuration and anteroposterior diameter
  Respiratory rate and depth
  Palpation to evaluate symmetry and tactile fremitus
  Percussion to evaluate tones and diaphragm excursion
  Auscultation to identify breath sound characteristics and adventitious sounds

Auscultation of other sounds

- **Heart and peripheral vascular system**

Location and characteristics of the apical impulse
Auscultation of S_1 and S_2 to note location, pitch, intensity, timing, splitting, systole, and diastole
Presence and characteristics of extra sounds, such as murmurs, clicks, snaps, S_3 and S_4
Jugular vein distention
Peripheral pulses: quality of pulses, bilaterally equal
Allen's test

- **Breasts and axillae**

Size and surface characteristics
Symmetry
Presence of masses, tenderness, discharge, dimpling
Presence of scars
Lymphatic assessment

- **Abdomen and gastrointestinal system**

Contour, visible aortic pulsations
Auscultation of all four quadrants to identify bowel sounds
Palpation of all four quadrants to identify organs, tenderness, masses
Costovertebral angle tenderness
Hernia

- **Female genitalia and reproductive system**

Characteristics of external genitalia
Speculum examination: note discharge, pain, surface characteristics of vagina, cervix, adnexa
Bimanual examination: note tenderness, masses, size of uterus and ovaries
Rectal examination

- **Male genitalia**

Characteristics of external genitalia
Palpation of penis and scrotum to note tenderness, discharge, lesions
Investigation of inguinal hernia to note swelling or tenderness

- **Anus, rectum, and prostate**

Prostate evaluation
Rectal examination

- **Musculoskeletal system**

Gait
Alignment of extremities and spine, symmetry of body

Joint evaluation
Muscle development, symmetry, and strength
Range of motion
Drawer test
McMurray's test

- **Neurologic system**

Mental status, thought processes, cognitive assessment
Cranial nerve assessment
Fine and gross motor function
Sensory evaluation
Reflexes

PART SIX

Reference Information

Abbreviations

A & P Anterior and posterior; auscultation and percussion
A & W Alive and well
abd Abdomen; abdominal
$\overline{\text{ac}}$ Before meals
ADL Activities of daily living
AJ Ankle jerk
AK Above knee
ANS Autonomic nervous system
AP Anteroposterior
bid Twice a day
BK Below knee
BP Blood pressure
BPH Benign prostatic hypertrophy
ENT Ear, nose, and throat
EOM Extraocular movement
FB Foreign body
FH Family history
FROM Full range of motion
FTT Failure to thrive
Fx Fracture
GB Gallbladder
GE Gastroesophageal
GI Gastrointestinal
GU Genitourinary
GYN Gynecologic
HA Headache
HCG Human chorionic gonadotropin

BS	Bowel sounds; breath sounds
c̄	With
CC	Chief complaint
CHD	Childhood disease; congenital heart disease; coronary heart disease
CHF	Congestive heart failure
CNS	Central nervous system
c/o	Complains of
COPD	Chronic obstructive pulmonary disease
CV	Cardiovascular
CVA	Costovertebral angle; cerebrovascular accident
CVP	Central venous pressure
Cx	Cervix
D & C	Dilation and curettage
D/C	Discontinued
DM	Diabetes mellitus
DOB	Date of birth
DOE	Dyspnea on exertion
DTRs	Deep tendon reflexes
DUB	Dysfunctional uterine bleeding
Dx	Diagnosis
ECG, EKG	Electrocardiogram; electrocardiograph
EENT	Eye, ear, nose, and throat
HEENT	Head, eyes, ears, nose, and throat
HOPI	History of present illness
HPI	History of present illness
Hx	History
ICS	Intercostal space
IOP	Intraocular pressure
IUD	Intrauterine device
IV	Intravenous
JVP	Jugular venous pressure
KJ	Knee jerk
KUB	Kidneys, ureters, and bladder
lat	Lateral
LCM	Left costal margin
LE	Lower extremities
LLL	Left lower lobe (lung)
LLQ	Left lower quadrant (abdomen)
LMD	Local medical doctor
LMP	Last menstrual period
LOC	Loss of consciousness; level of consciousness
LS	Lumbosacral; lumbar spine
LSB	Left sternal border
LUL	Left upper lobe (lung)
LUQ	Left upper quadrant (abdomen)
M	Murmur

Continued

Abbreviations—*Cont.*

MAL	Midaxillary line
MCL	Midclavicular line
MGF	Maternal grandfather
MGM	Maternal grandmother
MSL	Midsternal line
MVA	Motor vehicle accident
N & T	Nose and throat
N & V	Nausea and vomiting
NA	No answer; not applicable
NKA	No known allergies
NPO	Nothing by mouth
NSR	Normal sinus rhythm
OD	Oculus dexter; right eye
OM	Otitis media
OS	Oculus sinister; left eye
OTC	Over the counter
prn	As necessary
Pt	Patient
PVC	Premature ventricular contraction
q	Every
qd	Every day
qh	Every hour
qod	Every other day
RCM	Right costal margin
REM	Rapid eye movement
RLL	Right lower lobe (lung)
RLQ	Right lower quadrant (abdomen)
RML	Right middle lobe (lung)
ROM	Range of motion
ROS	Review of systems
RSB	Right sternal border
RUL	Right upper lobe (lung)

OU	Oculus uterque; each eye
$\bar{p}$	After
P & A	Percussion and auscultation
$\overline{pc}$	After meals
PE	Physical examination
PERRLA	Pupils equal, round, react to light and accommodation
PGF	Paternal grandfather
PGM	Paternal grandmother
PI	Present illness
PID	Pelvic inflammatory disease
PMH	Past medical history
PMI	Point of maximum impulse; point of maximum intensity
PMS	Premenstrual syndrome
RUQ	Right upper quadrant (abdomen)
$\bar{s}$	Without
SCM	Sternocleidomastoid
SQ	Subcutaneous
Sx	Symptoms
T & A	Tonsillectomy and adenoidectomy
TM	Tympanic membrane
TPR	Temperature, pulse, and respiration
UE	Upper extremities
URI	Upper respiratory infection
UTI	Urinary tract infection
WD	Well developed
WN	Well nourished
x	Times; by (size)

CONVERSION TABLES

Length

IN	CM	CM	IN
1	2.54	1	0.4
2	5.08	2	0.8
4	10.16	3	1.2
6	15.24	4	1.6
8	20.32	5	2.0
10	25.40	6	2.4
20	50.80	8	3.1
30	76.20	10	3.9
40	101.60	20	7.9
50	127.00	30	11.8
60	152.40	40	15.7
70	177.80	50	19.7
80	203.20	60	23.6
90	228.60	70	27.6
100	254.00	80	31.5
150	381.00	90	35.4
200	508.00	100	39.4

1 in = 2.54 cm
1 cm = 0.3937 in

Weight

LB	KG	KG	LB
1	0.5	1	2.2
2	0.9	2	4.4
4	1.8	3	6.6
6	2.7	4	8.8
8	3.6	5	11.0
10	4.5	6	13.2
20	9.1	8	17.6
30	13.6	10	22
40	18.2	20	44
50	22.7	30	66
60	27.3	40	88
70	31.8	50	110
80	36.4	60	132
90	40.9	70	154
100	45.4	80	176
150	66.2	90	198
200	90.8	100	220

1 lb = 0.454 kg
1 kg = 2.204 lb

Temperature

Fahrenheit and Celsius Equivalents: Body Temperature Range

F°	C°	F°	C°	F°	C°	F°	C°	F°	C°
9.04	34.44	97.0	36.11	100.0	37.78	103.0	39.44	106.0	41.11
94.2	34.56	97.2	36.22	100.2	37.89	103.2	39.56	106.2	41.22
94.4	34.67	97.4	36.33	100.4	38.00	103.4	39.67	106.4	41.33
94.6	34.78	97.6	36.44	100.6	38.11	103.6	39.78	106.6	41.44
94.8	34.89	97.8	36.56	100.8	38.22	103.8	39.89	106.8	41.56
95.0	35.00	98.0	36.67	101.0	38.33	104.0	40.00	107.0	41.67
95.2	35.11	98.2	36.78	101.2	38.44	104.2	40.11	107.2	41.78
95.4	35.22	98.4	36.89	101.4	38.56	104.4	40.22	107.4	41.89
95.6	35.33	98.6	37.00	101.6	38.67	104.6	40.33	107.6	42.00
95.8	35.44	98.8	37.11	101.8	38.78	104.8	40.44	107.8	42.11
96.0	35.56	99.0	37.22	102.0	38.89	105.0	40.56	108.0	42.22
96.2	35.67	99.2	37.33	102.2	39.00	105.2	40.67		
96.4	35.78	99.4	37.44	102.4	39.11	105.4	40.78		
96.6	35.89	99.6	37.56	102.6	39.22	105.6	40.89		
96.8	36.00	99.8	37.67	102.8	39.33	105.8	41.00		

To convert Centigrade or Celsius degrees to Fahrenheit degrees: multiply the number of Centigrade degrees by $9/5$ and add 32 to the result. To convert Fahrenheit degrees to Centigrade degrees: Subtract 32 from the number of Fahrenheit degrees and multiply the difference by $5/9$.

Height and Weight

			Men (indoor clothing*)					
			Small frame		Medium frame		Large frame	
Feet	Inches	Cm	Pounds	Kilograms	Pounds	Kilograms	Pounds	Kilograms
5	1	154.9	128-134	58.2-60.9	131-141	59.5-64.1	138-150	62.7-68.2
5	2	157.5	130-136	59.1-61.8	133-143	60.4-65.0	140-153	63.6-69.5
5	3	160.0	132-138	60.0-62.7	135-145	61.4-65.9	142-156	64.5-70.9
5	4	162.6	134-140	60.9-63.6	137-148	62.3-67.2	144-160	65.5-72.7
5	5	165.1	136-142	61.8-64.5	139-151	63.2-68.6	146-164	66.4-74.5
5	6	167.6	138-145	62.7-65.9	142-154	64.5-70.0	149-168	67.7-76.4
5	7	170.2	140-148	63.6-67.2	145-157	65.9-71.4	152-172	69.1-78.2
5	8	172.7	142-151	64.5-68.6	148-160	67.2-72.7	155-176	70.5-80.0
5	9	175.3	144-154	65.5-70.0	151-153	68.6-74.1	158-180	71.8-81.8
5	10	177.8	146-157	66.4-71.4	154-166	70.0-75.5	161-184	73.2-83.6
5	11	180.3	149-160	67.7-72.7	157-170	71.4-77.3	164-188	74.5-85.5
6	0	182.9	152-164	69.1-74.5	160-174	72.7-79.1	168-192	76.4-87.3
6	1	185.4	155-168	70.5-76.4	164-178	74.5-80.9	172-197	78.2-89.5
6	2	188.0	158-172	71.8-78.2	167-182	75.9-82.7	176-202	80.0-91.8
6	3	190.5	162-176	73.6-80.0	171-187	77.7-85.0	181-207	82.3-94.1

*Allow 5 pounds.

			Women (indoor clothing*)					
			Small frame		Medium frame		Large frame	
Feet	**Inches**	**Cm**	**Pounds**	**Kilograms**	**Pounds**	**Kilograms**	**Pounds**	**Kilograms**
4	9	144.8	102-111	46.4-50.0	109-121	49.5-55.0	118-131	53.6-59.5
4	10	147.3	103-113	46.8-51.4	111-123	50.0-55.9	120-134	54.5-60.9
4	11	149.9	104-115	47.3-52.3	113-126	51.4-57.2	122-137	55.5-62.3
5	0	152.4	106-118	48.2-53.6	115-129	52.3-58.6	125-140	56.8-63.6
5	1	154.9	108-121	49.1-55.0	118-132	53.6-60.0	128-143	58.2-65.0
5	2	157.5	111-124	50.5-56.4	121-135	55.0-61.4	131-147	59.5-66.8
5	3	160.0	114-127	51.8-57.7	124-138	56.4-62.7	134-151	60.9-68.6
5	4	162.6	117-130	53.2-59.0	127-141	57.7-64.1	137-155	62.3-70.5
5	5	165.1	120-133	54.5-60.5	130-144	59.0-65.5	140-159	63.6-72.3
5	6	167.6	123-136	55.9-61.8	133-147	60.5-66.8	143-163	65.0-74.1
5	7	170.2	126-139	57.3-63.2	136-150	61.8-68.2	146-167	66.4-75.9
5	8	172.7	129-142	58.6-64.5	139-153	63.2-69.5	149-170	67.7-77.3
5	9	175.3	132-145	60.0-65.9	142-156	64.6-70.9	152-173	69.1-78.6
5	10	177.8	135-148	61.4-67.3	145-159	65.9-72.3	155-176	70.5-80.0
5	11	180.3	138-151	62.7-73.6	148-162	67.3-73.6	158-179	71.8-81.4

*Allow 3 pounds.

The weights presented are those associated with the lowest mortality. They are not necessarily the weights at which people are healthiest, perform their jobs optimally, or even look their best. Three weight ranges were determined for each sex on each size and attributed to a small, medium, or large frame.

These tables correct the 1983 Metropolitan tables to height without shoe heels.

BODY MASS INDEX

Many professionals believe the body mass index (BMI) is a more objective indicator of the presence of obesity than the life insurance height and weight tables. Calculate BMI as follows:

$$\text{BMI} = \frac{\text{Weight (kg)}}{\text{Height (m}^2\text{)}}$$

IMMUNIZATION SCHEDULES

Schedule for Children Born in the United States*

Recommended Age†	Immunization(s)‡	Comments
Birth	HBV§	
1-2 months	HBV§	
2 months	DTP, Hib, OPV	DTP and OPV can be initiated as early as 4 weeks after birth in areas of high endemicity or during outbreaks.
4 months	DTP, Hib, OPV	2-month interval (minimum of 6 weeks) recommended for OPV
6 months	DTP, (Hib)‖	
6-18 months	HBV,§ OPV	MMR should be given at 12 months of age in high-risk areas; if indicated, tuberculin testing may be done at the same visit.
12-15 months	Hib, MMR	
15-18 months	DTaP or DTP	The fourth dose of diphtheria-tetanus-pertussis vaccine should

		be given 6 to 12 months after the third dose of DTP and may be given as early as 12 months of age, provided that the interval between doses 3 and 4 is at least 6 months and DTP is given; DTaP is not currently licensed for use in children younger than 15 months of age.
4-6 years	DTaP or DTP, OPV	DTaP or DTP and OPV should be given at or before school entry; DTP or DTaP should not be given at or after the seventh birthday.
11-12 years	MMR	MMR should be given at entry to middle school or junior high school unless 2 doses were given after the first birthday.
14-16 years	Td	Repeat every 10 years throughout life.

Modified from American Academy of Pediatrics, Committee on Infectious Diseases: *1994 Red Book: report of the Committee on Infectious Diseases,* ed 23, Elk Grove Village, Ill, 1994.

*Table is not completely consistent with all package inserts. For products used, also consult manufacturer's package insert for instructions on storage, handling, dosage, and administration. Biologics prepared by different manufacturers may vary, and package inserts of the same manufacturer may change from time to time. Therefore the practitioner should be aware of the contents of the current package insert.

†These recommended ages should not be construed as absolute. For example, 2 months can be 6 to 10 weeks. However, MMR usually should not be given to children younger than 12 months of age. If measles vaccination is indicated, monovalent measles vaccine is recommended, and MMR should be given subsequently at 12 to 15 months of age.

‡Vaccine abbreviations: *HBV,* Hepatitis B virus vaccine; *DTP,* diphtheria and tetanus toxoids and pertussis vaccine; *DTaP,* diphtheria and tetanus toxoids and acellular pertussis vaccine; *Hib,* Haemophilus influenzae type b conjugate vaccine; *OPV,* oral poliovirus vaccine (containing attenuated poliovirus types 1, 2, and 3); *MMR,* live measles, mumps, and rubella viruses vaccine; *Td,* adult tetanus toxoid (full dose) and diphtheria toxoid (reduced dose), for children ≥ 7 years and adults.

§An acceptable alternative to minimize the number of visits for immunizing infants of HBsAg-negative mothers is to administer dose 1 at 0 to 2 months, dose 2 at 4 months, and dose 3 at 6 to 18 months of age.

||Hib; dose 3 of Hib is not indicated if the product for doses 1 and 2 was PedvaxHIB (PRP-OMP).

Schedule for Children Not Immunized in the First Year of Life in the United States

Recommended time/age	Immunization(s)*,†	Comments
Younger than 7 years		
First visit	DTP, Hib, HBV, MMR, OPV	If indicated, tuberculin testing may be done at same visit. If child is 5 years of age or older, Hib is not indicated.
Interval after first visit:		
1 month	DTP, HBV	OPV may be given if accelerated poliomyelitis vaccination is necessary, such as for travelers to areas where polio is endemic.
2 months	DTP, Hib, OPV	Second dose of Hib is indicated only in children whose first dose was received when younger than 15 months of age.
≥ 8 months	DTP or DTaP‡, HBV, OPV	OPV is not given if the third dose was given earlier.
4-6 years (at or before school entry)	DTP or DTaP,‡ OPV	DTP or DTaP is not necessary if the fourth dose was given after the fourth birthday; OPV is not necessary if the third dose was given after the fourth birthday.
11-12 years	MMR	MMR should be given at entry to middle school or junior high school.
10 years later	Td	Repeat every 10 years throughout life.
7 years and older§,‖		
First visit	HBV,¶ OPV, MMR, Td	

Interval after first visit:		
2 months	HBV,¶ OPV, Td	OPV may also be given 1 month after the first visit if accelerated poliomyelitis vaccination is necessary.
8-14 months	HBV,¶ OPV, Td	OPV is not given if the third dose was given earlier.
11-12 years	MMR	MMR should be given at entry to middle school or junior high school.
10 years later	Td	Repeat every 10 years throughout life.

Modified from Wong DL: *Nursing care of infants and children,* ed 5, St Louis, 1995, Mosby.

*If all needed vaccines cannot be administered simultaneously, priority should be given to protecting the child against those diseases that pose the greatest immediate risk. In the United States these diseases for children younger than 2 years usually are measles and Haemophilus influenzae type b infection; for children older than 7 years, they are measles, mumps, and rubella (MMR).

†DTP or DTaP, HBV, Hib, MMR, and OPV can be given simultaneously at separate sites if failure of the patient to return for future immunizations is a concern.

‡DTaP is not currently licensed for use in children younger than 15 months of age and is not recommended for primary immunization (i.e., first 3 doses) at any age.

§If person is 18 years or older, routine poliovirus vaccination is not indicated in the United States.

||Minimal interval between doses of MMR is 1 month.

¶Priority should be given to hepatitis B immunization of adolescents.

CREDITS

Barkauskas VH et al: *Health and physical assessment,* St Louis, 1994, Mosby.

Chipps EM, Clanin NJ, Campbell VG: *Neurologic disorders,* St Louis, 1992, Mosby.

Folstein M et al: The meaning of cognitive impairment in the elderly, *J Am Geriatr Soc* 33(4):228, 1985.

Miyasaki-Ching CM: *Chasteen's essentials of clinical dental assisting,* ed 5, St Louis, 1997, Mosby.

Mourad LA: *Orthopedic disorders,* St Louis, 1991, Mosby.

Seeley RR, Stephens TD, Tate P: *Anatomy and physiology,* St Louis, 1995, Mosby.

Seidel HM et al: *Mosby's guide to physical examination,* ed 3, St Louis, 1995, Mosby.

Tanner JM: *Growth at adolescence,* ed 2, Oxford, England, 1962, Blackwell Scientific Publications.

Thibodeau GA, Patton KT: *Structure and function of the body,* ed 10, St Louis, 1997, Mosby.

Thompson JM et al: *Mosby's clinical nursing,* ed 3, St Louis, 1992, Mosby.

INDEX

A

B

C

D

E

H

I

N

O

P

Q

R

U

V

W

X

Y

Z